UNWANTED HAIR
AND HIRSUTISM

A BOOK FOR WOMEN

UNWANTED HAIR
AND HIRSUTISM
A BOOK FOR WOMEN

🍃 YOUR HEALTH PRESS

Alison Amoroso, M.Ed.

Unwanted Hair and Hirsutism: A Book for Women
First published by Your Health Press in association with Trafford Publishing.

Cover and Text Design: 729design
Cover Photo: ©iStockphoto

Important Notice:
The purpose of this book is to educate. It is sold with the understanding that the author and publisher shall have neither liability nor responsibility for any injury caused or alleged to be caused directly or indirectly by the information contained in this book. While every effort has been made to ensure its accuracy, the book's contents should not be construed as medical advice. Each person's health needs are unique. To obtain recommendations appropriate to your particular situation, please consult a qualified health care provider.

Order this book online at www.trafford.com
or email orders@trafford.com

Most Trafford titles are also available at major online book retailers.

© Copyright 2009 Alison Amoroso, M.Ed. and Your Health Press
All rights reserved. No part of this publication may be reproduced, stored in a retrieval system, or transmitted, in any form or by any means, electronic, mechanical, photocopying, recording, or otherwise, without the written prior permission of the author.
Note for Librarians: A cataloguing record for this book is available from Library and Archives Canada at www.collectionscanada.ca/amicus/index-e.html

Printed in Victoria, BC, Canada.

ISBN: 978-1-4269-2218-3

Library of Congress Control Number: 2009940588

Our mission is to efficiently provide the world's finest, most comprehensive book publishing service, enabling every author to experience success. To find out how to publish your book, your way, and have it available worldwide, visit us online at www.trafford.com

Trafford rev. 11/02/09

www.trafford.com
North America & international
toll-free: 1 888 232 4444 (USA & Canada)
phone: 250 383 6864 ♦ fax: 812 355 4082

OTHER *YOUR HEALTH PRESS* TITLES

The Frequent Fiber Cookbook: Easy and Delicious Recipes and Tips for People on a High Fiber Diet by Norene Gilletz and Mandy Erikson (2009)

Women and Alopecia: Managing Unexplained Hair Loss by L. Lee Culvert (2009)

Stopping Cancer at the Source: The Primary Prevention of Cancer, 2nd edition by M. Sara Rosenthal, Ph.D. (2008)

The PCOS Diet Cookbook: Delicious Recipes and Tips for Women with PCOS on the Low GI Diet by Nadir R. Farid, M.D. and Norene Gilletz (2007)

Coping with Molar Pregnancy and Choriocarcinoma by Tara Johnson and Meredith Schwartz (2007)

Preventing Menopause: How to Stop Menopause Before It Starts by Beth Rosenshein (2006)

Living Well with Celiac Disease: Abundance Beyond Wheat and Gluten, 2nd edition by Claudine Crangle (2006)

The Low-Iodine Diet Cookbook: Easy and Delicious Recipes and Tips for Thyroid Cancer Patients by Norene Gilletz (2005)

Menopause Before 40: Coping with Premature Ovarian Failure by Karin Banerd (2004)

Healing Injuries the Natural Way: How to Mend Bones, Muscles, Tendons & More by Michelle Cook (2004)

Thyroid Eye Disease: Understanding Graves' Ophthalmopathy by Elaine A. Moore (2003)

Living Well with an Ostomy by Elizabeth Rayson (2003)

The Thyroid Cancer Book, 2nd edition by M. Sara Rosenthal, Ph.D. (2003)

ACKNOWLEGMENTS

Many thanks to M. Sara Rosenthal, the dedicated publisher with a keen sense of how to help women by intertwining scientific knowledge and cultural experience. She asked me to write this book without knowing that I was one of many woman who hated my hair and struggled with it most of my life. I learned a lot about my own biology while researching and writing the book, and am grateful for the opportunity. I am also grateful to my husband, Robert Zegarra Fernandez-Baca, who doesn't see me through a hair "lens" and for his patience while I wrote this book. A big thank-you hug to my sister Cathy and friend Beckie McCuen, who helped me enormously by giving me the time to write and research while they watched Alisia. Many thanks to Debbie Liehs for her expert copyediting skills. And many, many thanks to the women who shared their own experiences with me in the heartfelt quotes and stories. I am also grateful to Patsy Kirby and Judy Adams for sharing their technical expertise with me.

TABLE OF CONTENTS

Introduction: If I Knew Then What I Know Now ... 12

Chapter 1. Don't Tweeze That Stray Hair! ... 15
Why Yanking Doesn't Work
   Why Is There Less Hair?
   Why Yanking Destroys Your Hair
Getting Rid of the Stray Hair You Hate
Changing Trends

Chapter 2. Our Hair ... 20
The Hair We Don't Want
All Humans Have Hair
   Why Is Hair Necessary?
   The Three Types of Hair
Hair Roots
Hair Growth Stages
   What Stage Is My Hair In?
Body Hair Transformed: From Vellus to Terminal Hair
   How It Happens
   Skin Interactions
   Terminal Hair: Dark, Coarse Hair
Talking to Your Adolescent Girl

Chapter 3. Hirsuitism: Too Much Hair ... 37
Types of Hair Growth That Qualify as Hirsutism
What Is Hirsutism?
What Is Hypertrichosis?
Diagnosing Hirsutism
Consulting a Doctor
   Finding a Trained Doctor
Common Causes of Hirsutism
   Polycystic Ovarian Syndrome
   Recreational Steroid Use
   Cushing's Syndrome

Drug Side Effects
  Insulin Resistance and Type 2 Diabetes
  Rare Endocrine Disorders
  Obesity
  Stress
  Tumors
  Related Symptoms

Chapter 4. Treatments for Hirsutism ... 56
Cosmetic Hair Removal
Hormone and Pharmacological Treatments
  Pregnancy
  Oral Contraceptives
  Antiandrogen Therapy
  Insulin-Lowering Drugs
  Glucocorticoid Therapy
  GnRH Agonists
  Stress Treatment
  Obesity Treatment
  Topical Skin Cream
  Other Treatments

Chapter 5. Polycystic Ovarian Syndrome: The Most Common Cause of Hirsutism ... 71
Possible Symptoms of PCOS
Associated Health Risks
  Changes in the Ovaries
Diagnosing PCOS
Causes of PCOS
The Role Genes Play in PCOS
The Role Insulin Plays in PCOS
Managing PCOS
  Exercise and Stress Reduction
  Eating the Low Glycemic Index Way
  The First Step to Eating Well
  Drug Therapies

Chapter 6. Hair: What Stimulates It and What Kills It ... 85
Real Women Grow Hair

Chapter 7. Hair Removal Methods ... 89
Shaving
    Cost and Convenience
Trimmers and Grooming Kits
Laser Razor
Tweezing
Electric Tweezers
    Cost and Convenience
Epilators
Hair Removal Cream
    Cost and Convenience
Growth-Inhibiting Cream
    Vaniqua
Bleaching Cream
    Cost and Convenience
Friction
    Cost and Convenience
Body Sugaring
Threading
    Cost and Convenience
Waxing
    Cost and Convenience
Home Electrolysis Kits
Miscellaneous Hair Removal Products and Scams
Summary of Electrolysis and Laser Treatment
    Electrolysis versus Laser Treatment

Chapter 8. Hair Removal by Body Part ... 108
Eyebrow Shaping
    Eyebrow Waxing at Nail Salons
    Cost and Convenience
Nose and Ear Hair
    Cost and Convenience

Toes, Belly Button/Happy Trail, Fingers
Bikini Area and Inner Thighs
Face
Neck, Back, and Torso

Chapter 9. Removing Pubic Hair ... 118
Benefits of Pubic Hair
Which Method Is Best?
   Hygiene Precautions for Brazilian Waxing
How to Avoid Vaginal Infections
   Vulvitis
   Yeast Infections
Women Who Should Not Remove Their Pubic Hair

Chapter 10. Electrolysis: What You Need to Know ... 125
A Brief History of Electrolysis
The Pain Myth
Safety Concerns
Aftercare
Timing Is Everything
Cost and Convenience
Setting Up a Consultation
   Finding a Qualified Provider
   What to Ask a Potential Electrologist
Credentials and Licensing Are Everything

Chapter 11. Laser Hair Removal: What You Need to Know ... 138
How Laser Hair Removal Works
Is Laser Hair Removal Right for You?
   Is Enough Ever Enough?
A Brief History of Laser Hair Removal
Preparation
Safety Concerns
Aftercare
Cost and Convenience
Setting Up a Consultation

Credentials and Regulations Are Everything
    Finding a Qualified Provider

Chapter 12. Protecting Yourself from Skin Damage: Risks and Regulations ... 149
Spas, Salons, and Medical Centers
Laser Treatments
    Is Laser Treatment Experimental Therapy?
Disclosure Statements

Chapter 13. Improving Your Body Image—Hair and All ... 152
Withstanding Cultural Influences
Body Hair Activism
    The Personal
    The Cultural
    The Political
    The Personal Is Political

Appendix A ... 159
Can't Stop Obsessing

Appendix B ... 161
Common Prescription Drugs That May Cause Hair Growth

Appendix C ... 163
Oral Contraception
Estrogen versus Progestin: Side Effects
Different Bodies Need Different Oral Contraceptives

Bibliography ... 165

Index ... 170

INTRODUCTION: IF I KNEW THEN WHAT I KNOW NOW

When I was a teenager, my grandmother often asked me why I shaved the hair on my legs. Her question seemed silly to me. Why wouldn't I? Was there a choice?

She then showed me her legs, which I wasn't accustomed to seeing. She was an old lady, after all! Her hair was soft, fine, and lay down all by itself. It was the color of the hair on her head—or must have been before she was gray. She said, "See—if you don't shave, then your legs would look like this instead of like yours." Mine were stubbly, the hair was dark and coarse, and I had a few ingrown hairs that drove me crazy.

But it was too late. I was in the hair removal cycle, as was virtually every other postpubescent woman in the United States. By my late teens, I was thoroughly involved in critiquing myself and other young women who "allowed" a hair to show on their calves or underarms, and I was investing time and money in trying to improve my hair removal techniques (and dealing with the pain). I didn't know that this was a losing battle for a woman descended from generations of women from the Mediterranean—yes, I have dark, coarse hair. Like my poor mother whom my siblings and I teased mercilessly, my hair seems to grow back almost immediately after I remove it.

When did this cultural change begin? When did women start to not only remove their body hair, but become obsessed about it at an early age? Clearly sometime after the 1930s, when my grandmother was a young, fashionable woman working in Manhattan. Hair is part of our anatomy, after all, and an integral part of our body.

History, however, is not the subject of this book, managing our current cultural preoccupation to remove hair is. (For an interesting analysis of the historical and cultural effects on women in the early part of the last century, particularly the backlash against women when they began organizing for legal rights, read the chapter on body image in *Our Bodies, Ourselves: A New Edition for a New Era*.)

There are many levels of hair quantity and texture, not to mention shades of color that cause hair to show more or less prominently. Of course, during certain stages of women's menstrual cycle, some hair becomes darker (pigment actually changes) and more prominent than it normally is, causing much consternation around this monthly event.

For many women, hormonal imbalances caused by certain medical disorders or medications come with the extra burden of finding their hair growing faster or finding it growing in the same places as it does for men (called male-pattern growth). Our culture's disdain for women with excessive body hair is particularly difficult for women with hair growth in areas we associate with male bodies. This condition is called *hirsutism*. In this book, I will make a special effort to address concerns for dealing with unwanted hair if you have hirsutism or you think you may have it.

It is strange to think that hair has taken on a defining role for women, whether it is hair on our head, the shape of our eyebrows, or the equation that hairlessness is sexy; after all, we are human, and humans have hair on every body part except for three areas (the palms of our hands, the soles of our feet, and our lips). So weren't women sexy before razors were placed into cheap, plastic containers?

Sure, there are historical accounts about people trying to get rid of their hair over the centuries, but these are merely anecdotes that were probably only practiced by small subsets of people. For example, Cleopatra was said to use some sort of hair removal process; royalty in every culture does many things the rest of us do not. And perhaps if you had hirsutism in any century, you would feel pressured to get rid of some of the hair, too.

There are just as many anecdotes about a woman's body hair being desirable. For instance, in ancient India, the thin line of dark hair on the upper abdomen, called the *romaraji*, was considered to be a mark of great beauty. So don't let anyone con you into thinking that women since antiquity have been dilapidating and therefore it must be normal; even well-meaning books and Web sites that highlight famous hair removers in history omit the cultures that appreciate female anatomy or celebrate anomalies.

However, the cultural pressure for women to rid themselves of hair (which is now spreading to men) is far and wide. There are many theories about power and womanhood and why hairlessness is so important in our culture right now, which are worth exploring the "root" of this mind-set. And who knows, perhaps learning about these theories will inspire you to become an activist.

Unwanted Hair and Hirsutism

No matter what your ethnic makeup, you likely feel pressure to get rid of any body or facial hair you were born with. Women who have descended from or emigrated from parts of the world that produce lots of hair, especially dark hair, and women with hirsutism have a particularly hard route to attain the hairless ideal that permeates U.S. culture.

Certainly, most of the world never adopted the U.S. ideal or a similar version of it. How happy I was to travel to western Europe, where the citizens are considered our peers. Here were competent, self-confident, beautiful women with lots of body hair! Okay, so many are light skinned and fair haired, but they just don't worry about their hair. And, surprise! Men don't shun them. They have boyfriends, marry, and are employed. Women who travel out of the United States have this experience all over the world, often visiting the place of their ancestors and seeing women who hold their head up high, facial hair and all.

Perhaps now that the United States has more fair immigration policies than it once did, our melting pot will turn our culture around, and women will be respected for all of our anatomy. We are already witnessing changes. Take *Ugly Betty*, the Colombian television show adapted for a U.S. audience, for example. This runaway hit speaks to all women, thick eyebrows and all, not just Latinas. And it is precisely because Betty has thick eyebrows and looks like a real woman—and is attractive the way she is—that women love the show.

But until the time comes when women are appreciated for all of our anatomy, many of us have to cope daily or weekly with ridding ourselves of hair. And that is what this book is about.

The feminist adage that "the personal is political" has never been truer when it comes to women and unwanted hair. For the purposes of this book, the phrase means that within one woman's story and struggles with unwanted hair, you can find all women's stories and struggles.

If every woman knew at age twelve the information in this book, she could save herself endless "woman hours" of bleaching, plucking, breaking her skin, and picking at scabs in embarrassing places.

This book covers it all—from brows to toes. Discover why unwanted hair grows and the best ways to treat it or remove it. Find detailed information on all the removal methods out there, including electrolysis and laser treatment. Most important, learn what not to do, because many methods actually worsen the problem and encourage hair growth.

CHAPTER 1

DON'T TWEEZE THAT STRAY HAIR!

Yes, it's true. Don't do it. Don't pluck out the hair you hate under your belly button, on your big toe, sticking out of your chin, or any other place you don't want it. This hair is not the same as your eyebrow hair; you're not going to shape your happy trail.

Here's why.

When you tweeze your hair with tweezers, your fingernails, your teeth, or any other device that grips your hair and yanks it out, you are actually making the future hair that grows from that spot stronger. Soon another hair will take its place, and it will be tougher than the one you yanked out. You probably thought if you yanked the hair hard enough and pulled out the little black ball at the base, called a bulb, that you had removed the root once and for all. Unfortunately, that is not the case.

By pulling it out, you may also be causing the next hairs that grow from that follicle to be coarser and darker, especially after repeated plucking. And that is not what you want. The same thing goes for waxing, sugaring, threading, stringing, or electronic devices that pull out your hair. All of these procedures can make your hair grow back stronger, coarser, and darker. The technical word for the removal of hair is *epilation*.

None of these removal techniques will prevent that hair from growing back in that same spot. Horrors! It looks like you got the root, right? Whatever is at the end looks like a root, but your body is smarter than that. Your cells just make another hair within the exact same hair follicle.

There are only three ways to permanently get rid of a hair from growing in a particular spot. One is by growing older and outliving the life of that hair follicle. Another method is electrolysis. And the third way to permanently remove a hair is by damaging the follicle so that the hair growth cells stop regenerating, which can accidentally happen while yanking a hair or during laser hair removal. Other ways you may indirectly lose hair are caused by medications, stress, hormonal imbalance, and other physical disorders.

Hair grows from something akin to a seed, and pulling the root does not kill the seed, no matter how many times you pull. That hair follicle is programmed to grow hair a certain amount of times over the course of your lifetime and there is little you can do about it by plucking. (See chapter 2 for more information about how hair grows.) We all have about 5 million hair follicles covering our body, and about 100,000 alone cover the scalp.

WHY YANKING DOESN'T WORK

There is a reason why yanking, tweezing, waxing, sugaring, threading, stringing, and electronic devices that grip and pull out your hair don't work. These methods attack the skin, causing your body to send blood supplies to the area. The blood then nourishes the hair follicle and makes it stronger. Not only do these epilating methods irritate the skin; because the hair's function is to protect the skin, your body goes into defense mode. You have destroyed the first layer of defense—your hair—and the hair then must strengthen itself.

Yanking swaths of hair using waxing, sugaring, threading, stringing, or electronic devices pulls out the hair strands you see *and* the very fine, light hair called *vellus hair* that grows all over your body. You may call this hair peach fuzz. Yanking with these methods stimulates the hair follicles, and then the hair that does grow back—having been now strengthened—grows in coarser and darker than it was. So now you will see even more hair in the area you just yanked (the hair was always there but just not as noticeable). Yikes. This is surely not what you intended.

Not so, you say? Well, the reason you don't see a change after just a few waxings or threadings, or other epilation methods, is because it takes multiple attacks for the hair to become darker and coarser. Good news, indeed, if you are just getting started. If you intend to pull out your hair in the same area over time, now you know what to look forward to, or if you've been doing it, you may understand why it does not seem like you can stop.

Here's another problem: if you pluck a hair during its "resting phase," you will "wake up" its growing process. As a result, you will stimulate a hair back into its active growing phase, causing it to poke through your skin faster than it would have otherwise. If you leave that hair you hate alone, it will cycle through its growth phase and fall out on its own. It might bother you for a few days, but then it won't grow back for a while.

Why Is There Less Hair?

You may think tweezing or waxing is working because you notice that hair in that area is thinning out. Women will notice this after age thirty or so. This is because some hairs naturally have a shorter regrowth life than others, especially eyebrows. Eyebrows and eyelashes have the shortest life span of all hair, whereas the hair on your head has among the longest. Pubic hair is also relatively short-lived. But as these types of hair thin, you will likely start to notice hair coming out your nose or chin instead as you age.

Why Yanking Destroys Your Hair

So have you ever thought a hair was gone for good after a good tweeze?

In some cases, if you yank out a hair, scar tissue will form around the follicle area where the root was pulled (called *keloids*), preventing hair growth, which is why some women may notice less hair growth when they wax or sugar (but rarely do they notice it with tweezing).

Or it may look like you "killed" the hair because you've noticed less hair growth in that area. In reality, the hair growth cells in that follicle are not dead; the hair is just cycling through its growth phase and will reappear eventually only to taunt you again.

However, one outcome of tweezing, pulling, plucking, biting, or otherwise yanking hair out that is just as likely as forming scar tissue around the follicle, is that you may cause an ingrown hair or an infection of the hair shaft. This infection, called *folliculitis*, causes the hair to be blocked in its natural route and curl into your skin looking for another way out. Folliculitis resembles acne because it contains a pocket of pus. An ingrown hair is similar: the hair cuts back into the skin, often eventually finding a way out. Also, be careful not to pick at it, because that's a good way to cause an infection or scarring.

GETTING RID OF THE STRAY HAIR YOU HATE

So what's a girl to do about a few stray hairs?

A stray hair, or two or three, can be cut with sharp, fine scissors. You may have to shop at a specialty pharmacy for these scissors, but they are handy for other times you need to do close cutting. They are small with sharp edges and are meant to get close to the target. For more information about snipping stray hair whether or not you always have them, they come during particular parts of your menstrual cycle, or you keep discovering new ones as you age or experience menopause—see chapter 7.

Unwanted Hair and Hirsutism

Shaving blunts hair, making it look and feel coarser when the fine point of the hair strand is removed; therefore the shaved hairs may appear a little bushy. And who wants to go from a few stray hairs to bushy toes, for instance? Shaving also may be a dangerous alternative for a few stray hairs depending on where they are located (your breasts, for example).

Bleaching and hair removal cream is not as extreme as yanking a hair and there is little risk of ingrown hair and folliculitis, so these methods might work for some areas. They are also temporary because hair is designed to protect the skin from harsh elements, and when you irritate your skin with hot wax or chemicals your skin's response is to nourish the follicles with blood, increasing the hair growth. If you can live with the hair that is lighter in color and doesn't contrast with your skin too much, you might try bleach. Temporary removal techniques such as hair removal creams or laser treatment may be a solution in some situations (see chapters 7 and 10 for more information).

The only permanent solution to removing hair is electrolysis (see chapter 9). However, why spend all that money and time for a few hairs you can snip off once a month or so?

It is likely that you notice your body hair more during the time of your menstrual cycle, when the hair becomes darker. If that is the case, try to ignore the hair until your hormones cycle through and the color better fades into your skin. On the other hand, if it is the appropriate season, go outside and get a tan. Darker skin makes the hair less noticeable.

However, stray hairs are the least of many women's hair problems. For many of us, the hair above our lip, around our pubic area, or myriad other places drives us nuts. If you can't stop from worrying or obsessing about how your hair looks to you or others, see appendix A for some tips. Another solution may be to learn to accept your body and live with the hair you were born with. After reconditioning your mind, your hair won't bother you so much, and maybe you will even embrace it as you learn about your ethnic heritage and appreciate the amazing abilities of your body.

Over time, most women do learn to live with their hair. Perhaps other priorities push out our obsessions with our appearance, or we learn to like our hair. If you are young, this may be little consolation; except know that there is a good chance you won't feel as self-conscious as you get older. Throughout this book you will read the words of women who have changed their opinion about hair and their self-perception, for example,

Unwanted Hair and Hirsutism

I have come to appreciate my leg hair more. I'm also old enough now to be more confident with my dating partners vis-à-vis not worrying so much about what they think of my hairiness. —L.J.

CHANGING TRENDS

Even if you kind of like your hair or are used to it, many women feel compelled to get rid of it to fit in at work, their social circle, or to please their partner. In recent years, hairlessness has been touted as sexier or cleaner, as if the ability of hair to protect our bodies against dirt and germs has suddenly disappeared. No longer does the lion's mane capture the nation's attention as sexy, even for men, unless it is on one's head. The clean-shaven, preppy look seems to have taken over the nation's consciousness as ideal grooming, and now trends are moving toward men's hairlessness, too. Witness the painful scene in the *40-Year-Old Virgin* where Steve Carell is cowed into waxing his chest, or the increase in hair removal spas for men. Once in a while a female star emerges who actually has some of her eyebrows, or we'll see a male star with intact facial hair. However, these are entertainers; rarely do we see a newscaster, businessperson, or politician deviate from the norm.

There is also the false perception that a woman is more sexually potent when she is hairless. This perception is driven by the pornography industry, which has forcefully promoted the idea that breast augmentation equates with sexual prowess.

Unfortunately, there is a lack of serious attention paid to unwanted hair by girls' and women's health-care providers. Make no mistake: unwanted hair is a very serious problem for at least 10 percent of the female population. Hirsutism significantly contributes to lower self-esteem and a negative body image, which can predispose women to depression. Having good information about how to cope with unwanted hair can help empower more women and validate their experiences.

The rest of this book takes a look at the range of unwanted hair growth—including excessive hair growth—and some causes and treatments. It also describes how hair grows so you can fully understand how to get rid of it and perhaps learn to appreciate it. Hair truly is a remarkable part of our body.

CHAPTER 2

OUR HAIR

I was on the playground at recess during second grade wearing a short-sleeve top on one of the first nice days of spring. A girl asked me if I was a monkey. She said only animals have hair on their arms, not people. Up until that point, I had never noticed that I had hair on my arms. I was devastated. For years after that I worked on getting a tan as early in the season as I could, because when my skin was brown the hair would bleach blond and wouldn't be so noticeable (or ugly, I thought).
—C.F.

THE HAIR WE DON'T WANT

If you are reading this book, chances are you have a similar painful memory, or many years of dealing with angst about hair you don't like or want. This book uses the term *unwanted hair* to refer to hair growth on our body that is considered to be culturally unacceptable or unattractive. Unfortunately, the culture in the United States seems preoccupied with ridding us women of more and more hair, except on our head, where it is supposed to be full and healthy.

The color of unwanted hair is also key: the darker it is, the more visible it is, and therefore the more undesirable, according to societal norms. This distinction makes hair growth more of a problem for dark-haired women than for fair-haired women.

There is also a distinction between normal hair growth in undesirable areas (meaning, hair that is "supposed to be there") and abnormal hair growth in undesirable areas (meaning, hair that is "not supposed to be there"). Hair on the legs, arms, and underarm area, as well as fine hair on the upper lip and around the hairline on the sides of our face (the "sideburn" area), may be unwanted and undesirable, but it is perfectly normal. Thick, bushy eyebrows also fall into this category.

The fine hair on the upper lip or around the hairline may feel abnormal but it is not; it is merely visible. The next time you are in the company of a true blonde or a prepubescent girl, you may notice similar hair growth on her upper lip or hairline, but since this fine hair is light, it is not visible or stigmatizing. Caucasian women of Mediterranean (e.g., Italian, Greek, or Turkish) and Middle and Near Eastern origin (e.g., Pakistani, Persian, or Indian), typically are "blessed" with healthy hair growth in these areas.

In fact, in many other Western countries, women do not remove hair that is considered undesirable in the United States. In those countries, it is considered culturally acceptable to do nothing about hair on the legs, forearms, underarms, and upper lip, in addition to fine "sideburns." The few hairs around the nipples after puberty are considered normal, too.

Nordic and Anglo-Saxon European peoples, indigenous natives of North and South America, and African Americans have less hair than people from the Mediterranean region (men and women). East Asians have even less hair than Euro-Americans. Approximately one-third of all women who are not of Scandinavian or Asian descent have hair on their upper lip, around their nipples, or immediately outside of the pubic area. Therefore, contrary to what you may think, it is a large majority of women who *do* have hair in these areas.

If you are blessed with hair, too, but are trying to fit in or at least figure out what is considered normal, remember there is not one way. Aboriginal Ainus in Japan, for instance, show their long dark hair to prove they are members of the tribe. Therefore, if you are descended from peoples with a lot of hair and are blessed with thick hair on your head, you likely have thick hair in other places. However, if you are of Native American descent, for example, you likely have thick hair on your head, but not on the rest of your body. Women in our culture may like this but their brothers may not like having a bare chest.

If you have thick eyebrows, just think, you won't have to lament over their falling out when you are older and drawing them in with a pencil, making you afraid to go swimming or to sweat.

Learn to assess with skepticism the cultural norms you see among your peers or on television. Not only do customs change from year to year, but they change from town to town. What you may feel and see living in your neighborhood now may be completely different from what you may feel if you move to another area, or if you are a teenager and go away to college. Try to hang in there, expose yourself to other "normals," and not judge yourself too harshly.

Unwanted Hair and Hirsutism

What is important to understand is that there are many versions of normal, no matter what anyone tells you. One of the most famous contemporary examples of women celebrating their body with all its hair is Mexican artist Frida Kahlo, whose self-portraits illustrate her facial and body hair. So take a stand and define what is normal for you.

ALL HUMANS HAVE HAIR

The only places we're not supposed to grow hair are the palms of our hands, the soles of our feet, and our lips. Otherwise, human bodies are completely covered with hair, which we have to protect our skin and maintain our body temperature. In fact, all mammals have roughly the same hair biology.

The number of hair follicles on our bodies is predetermined at birth. No matter what you have done to your hair, or will do to it—no matter how many times you pull out a hair—you won't actually cause the numbers of hairs you have to increase or decrease. Even though we see more hair on men, they do not have more hair follicles on their body than do women. Both sexes have the same amount of hair follicles.

The number of hair follicles throughout anyone's body is genetically determined. What differs among ethnic groups is the rate at which hair grows (fastest for people whose ancestors came from the Mediterranean), the length it grows, the texture, the thickness of each strand, and the color. A full head of hair can come from a lot of follicles and/or thick hair strands. In general, Asian hair is thicker and more coarse than Caucasian and African-American hair, but it is less dense than that typically observed in Caucasians. On the scalp, Asians have between 90,000 and 120,000 follicles (although it is rarely this high). Caucasians have between 100,000 and 150,000 scalp hair follicles, with a range generally associated with hair color; blonds have the most and redheads the least.

You can, however, *cause* a hair to grow faster while you attempt to get rid of it. You can also damage the hair follicle and cause your skin to scar, which could be something else you wish to get rid of! Yanking a hair out causes both of these problems.

Under certain situations, hair can grow faster, darker, and longer than it should, or in places it typically grows for men but not for women in your ethnic group. This abnormally excessive hair growth is called *hirsutism* (pronounced her-SUIT-ism), a condition that is often caused by a hormonal imbalance or another medical disorder, which can usually be treated or that disappears when the stressor is removed. Women with hirsutism are described as being hirsute by medical professionals. A related condition is called hypertrichosis. It also results in excessive hair growth; however, it usually grows in nonsexual body parts. Hypertrichosis is a description for hair that generally grows faster, longer, and often darker than what is normal for the ethnic group from which one is descended. (See chapter 3 for more information.)

Another description of excess hair you might have heard about is called lanugo. Humans are born with it and it sheds soon after birth. This excess hair covers the body and is very soft and fine in texture. People with anorexia nervosa grow lanugo to keep their body warm. Their hormones are also imbalanced so the hair does not grow properly. Hair is necessary for the body to function, and in this case, one's body grows hair to mediate the damage anorexia is wreaking on it. Anorexia is a serious condition and one that requires professional help to treat. If you even suspect that your daughter is becoming anorexic, seek help immediately.

This book focuses primarily on unwanted hair and hirsutism, but let's first learn more about hair so you can be informed about how and why it grows. This knowledge can help you to make good decisions about how to get rid of hair on different parts of your body—if that is what you want—safely and effectively. Understanding how hair grows can alert you to the possibility you are stimulating your roots, and therefore your hair growth, by self-treating an unwanted hair problem. And that can start an endless, vicious cycle. Finally, understanding how amazing hair is may help you accept it on your own body and that of others.

Why Is Hair Necessary?

Hair's sole mission in life is to serve the skin. And there's no denying that skin is pretty important! Body hair is referred to as a *skin appendage* because it helps the skin—the body's largest organ—carry out its functions.

Our skin performs the following functions:
- Acts as a barrier between the internal organs and the external environment
- Protects us from the elements, such as chemicals, parasites, and organisms, as well as the sun

- Maintains our temperature control through perspiration or water absorption
- Helps our immune system respond to external chemicals or infections, such as *Staphylococcus* infections, some of which are becoming more and more common and infectious
- Gives us our tactile senses—our sensitivity to heat, cold, pressure, light, touch, itch, or pain; the epidermal cells have fine nerve endings scattered between them
- Secretes *sebum*, "skin oil," that lubricates all of the skin, including the scalp
- Makes us attractive socially and sexually (a healthy skin texture and scent is a sign of social and fertile health)
- Protects us further from the sun with melanocytes, which are pigment-producing cells (in hotter climates, skin is darker; in colder climates, it is lighter)

Other skin appendages besides hair include nails, sweat glands, sebaceous glands (the glands that secrete oils), and apocrine glands (the glands responsible for body odor, which apparently don't help human beings as much as they do other animals).

Hair is designed to protect and warm the skin. The hair is the protector of the skin; what does not destroy it, makes it stronger! In other words, if you stimulate a hair's roots by yanking it out, that hair will grow stronger rather than weaker.

The Three Types of Hair

We are all born with hair. It is part of being human (and a mammal). The first type does not stay with us long. It grows in the embryo stage and is the first hair we ever have. When we are born, it is called *lanugo hair*. Sometimes you can see it fall off a newborn, and new parents are warned about it lest they think something is wrong with their baby. It can be dark, but usually it is not. During the first year of life, the hair follicles change structurally into *vellus* hair, which covers our entire body, including our face, stomach, and shoulders. Vellus hair is typically soft, light, short, and fine in texture. The color, or lack thereof, is referred to as unpigmented.

The third category of hair is *terminal hair*. It is visible, dark, and coarse and it can be curly. It is longer and thicker than vellus hair. The hair follicle itself is longer and wider than in the other two types of hair. It grows in areas of our body that are generally reactive to hormones in our bloodstream. For example, pubic hair is kinky. Hair around the anus is associated with oil glands. The color of terminal hair is usually referred to as pigmented. The role of pigmentation is extremely important for certain types of removal techniques, especially for people with dark skin.

So when people say smooth as a baby's bottom, they don't mean hairless, because vellus hair is soft and fine in texture. If an advertisement uses the analogy of a baby's bottom to promote hair-removing techniques, the sales pitch is off base. Be forewarned that the company doesn't know much about hair!

Some terminal hair grows right from birth, such as the hair on the head, eyelashes, and eyebrows. Before we get into which hair grows when and where, let's take a look at how hair grows.

HAIR ROOTS

The hair is "rooted" in the *epidermis* (the outer layer of the skin). But a hair strand's root is not the same as a plant's root—contrary to popular belief, you can't pull it out and get rid of it once and for all. The cells that are responsible for the hair's growth remain as part of your tissues and keep growing more hair in that same spot unless those cells are killed, damaged to the point they can't produce any more, or stop producing hair due to aging or hormonal imbalances.

The *hair shaft* is the part of the hair we can see growing from our skin's surface, the epidermis. It is made from a protein called keratin, which is technically dead. Therefore, by cutting or shaving the dead hair shaft, you can't affect the hair's ability to grow. Hair is really just an outgrowth of the epidermis. In fact, both hair and skin are composed of keratin.

The hair shaft is produced inside the hair follicle, which is made up of two regions: the hair bulb and the midfollicle region.

- Sometimes the hair bulb is described as a sac. The hair bulb contains actively growing cells called *dermal papilla*, which are responsible for the hair's regrowth, and pigment-producing cells that are responsible for the hair's color.
- The midfollicle region is where actively growing cells die and harden into what we call hair.

Unwanted Hair and Hirsutism

The hair follicle can produce vellus hair (pale, fine, and short) and terminal hair (darker, coarser, longer, and larger). Which type the hair follicle produces depends on the chemical reactions in your body and your genes. There are also two types of hair follicles:

- Shallow hair follicles live in the *dermis*, a slightly deeper level of skin than the epidermis, which it supports. Our blood vessels and nerves are located in the dermis, as well as sweat and the oil-producing sebaceous glands.
- Larger, deeper hair follicles and sweat glands originate in the subcutaneous tissue layer, the layer of skin that lies beneath the dermis. (See figure 1.)

Figure 1. Negroid (Curly) Hair Follicle

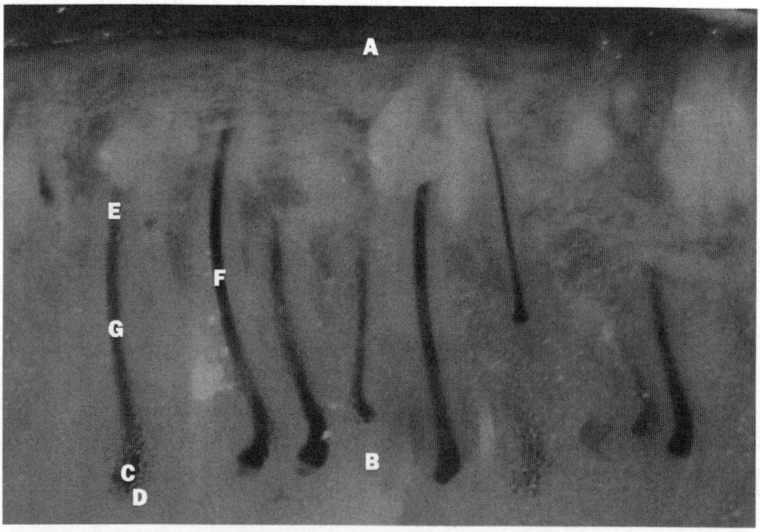

A. Epidermal layer of skin
B. Subcutaneous tissue layer of skin
C. Hair bulb
D. Dermal papilla
E. Hair shaft
F. Hair follicle (hair bulb plus hair shaft)
G. Midfollicle region

Photo Credit: Photomicrographs and many more are available from Prestige Electrolysis Supply, 1-800-783-7403, www.prestigeelec.com.

HAIR GROWTH STAGES

Removing a hair effectively depends on the growth stage it is in. During its life span, a hair goes through three distinct phases. Understanding these phases is important not only to choose an effective hair removal method but also to understand what is happening in your body and what to expect as you remove the hair. After a hair dies and sheds, another hair grows from the same follicle. The dermal papilla are most unique among cells in our body because they maintain the same regenerative properties in adults as they did during the embryonic stage of development. (In other words, most cells die as we age, but these cells continue to regenerate.)

The three phases of hair growth are called *anagen, catagen*, and *telogen*. These phases generally last a specific amount of time. For instance, the hair on our scalp grows longer than other hair because it has a longer growing phase. However, different body regions produce hair of different lengths, again depending on your ethnicity and life stage. The phases also can change depending on what you are doing to your body. For example, the resting stage can be shorter depending on medications you are taking, weight gain, steroid use, and medical conditions. Let us look at each phase.

Figure 2. Anagen Hair Follicles in Thin Slice of Human Scalp

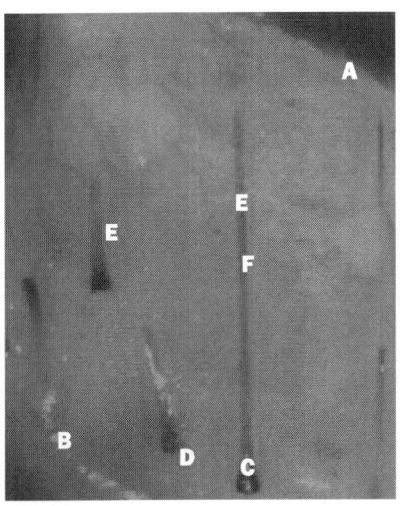

A. Epidermal layer of skin
B. Subcutaneous tissue layer of skin
C. Hair bulb
D. Dermal papilla
E. Hair shaft (hair bulb plus hair shaft
F. Hair follicle

Photo Credit: *Photomicrographs and many more are available from Prestige Electrolysis Supply, 1-800-783-7403, www.prestigeelec.com.*

Unwanted Hair and Hirsutism

Anagen
The anagen phase is the hair's active growth stage. It begins the moment the inactive hair follicle "comes to life" and descends to the papilla, which connects to the nourishment source—the blood supply. This stage ends when the dermal papilla ceases to nourish the hair, at which time the hair comes loose from the papilla.

In this phase, the cells in our hair follicles continuously make protein and keratin to promote the development and active growth of our hair shafts (see figure 1). At any point in time, 85 to 90 percent of hair is in the anagen phase, which can last from a few months up to six years.

Catagen
After the anagen phase, hair enters a transitional phase, called catagen, when chemical and structural changes within the hair follicle cause it to regress and stop growing.

During the catagen phase, the lower half of the follicle degenerates and the cells undergo a *retrograde morphogenic transformation*, which is a complete reversal of the growth process. Instead of the follicle reaching downward to the blood supply, it shrinks upward toward the surface of the skin.

Telogen
In the final part of the cycle, the telogen phase, the hair follicle shuts down and goes into resting mode. All that remains below the upper half of the follicle is a collection of hair germ cells from the outer root sheath and the dormant dermal papilla cells. At this stage the hair "hangs out" until it is shed and new growth begin. This phase can last up to one hundred days.

What Stage Is My Hair In?
At any given time, some of the hair will be in the growing stage, some in the resting stage, and some in the shedding stage; therefore, what you see at any time is not all of your hair, some is underneath your skin busily growing and ready to emerge. And, depending on your life stage, location on your body, or menstrual cycle, as well as how many times you are yanking it out, the next time it emerges it could grow in darker, or a vellus hair could change into a terminal hair.

However, just because you yank out a hair or two from your upper lip, chin, nose, or under your belly button, it doesn't mean the hair in those regions will change completely. Hair growth in humans is asynchronous, meaning that what is happening in each hair follicle is independent of surrounding follicles. This is also important to note for hair removal treatments such as cream and laser. If you treat a particular area, it will get rid of the hair strands that have emerged through your skin, but there are plenty more getting ready to pop up.

BODY HAIR TRANSFORMED: FROM VELLUS TO TERMINAL HAIR

My brother has Down syndrome. Going through puberty is difficult enough, but add the difficulty of understanding some things and puberty is even more complicated.

My brother went through a phase during which he began telling us that he wanted to grow up to be a woman. Transgender issues are something my family could negotiate and embrace, I am sure. But transgender issues on top of Down syndrome—well, I can say my parents had worries. As I was the psychology student of the family and consultant on all such topics, I was asked to help better understand my brother's desire to be a woman and to figure out ways to support him.

My first strategy was to talk about how exciting it was that he would soon be a man and not a boy anymore and how that change was very exiting. My brother disagreed, right away. Yet, as I spoke to my brother, it became clear that he did not think, as my sisters and I know, that being a woman often is not associated with a lot of perks. When asked (and my brother didn't), I note gender inequities in salary and the history of oppression as problems, for example.

Finally, it came out. My brother didn't want to be a man because he didn't like all the hair—the dark hair that was growing all over his body. He said if he became a woman, then he wouldn't have the hair. His problem would be solved. It was then that I had to tell him, "You know, we get the hair, too." He just looked at me, shocked and then said, "Where is it? I don't see it."

I then explained the art of shaving. I said he could shave, too, if he wanted. Given this new information, he decided to try being a man again. With shaving, he could have it all. —C.C.

Unwanted Hair and Hirsutism

As with the rest of our body, most of our hair also changes during puberty. Many of our light, soft vellus hairs are transformed into dark, coarse terminal hairs. This happens only in certain places on our body, but all women with normal sexual development experience their vellus hairs transforming into terminal hairs on their face, underarms, pubic area, inner thigh, and external genitalia. Most experience it also on their areolas, lower back, and buttocks.

The extent and amount of hair being transformed, its length and texture, and its growth rate are different for people with different ethnic backgrounds because it is controlled by our genes. So, for instance, you may have a lot of hair on the side of your face turning dark and long, and your friend doesn't, but generally this hair growth is a normal occurrence for people within your ethnic group. On the other hand, you may see razor stubble right away whereas a friend using the same type of razor doesn't get it for days. This deviation is one reason that hair removal products work so differently for different people.

How It Happens

Your hair changes from vellus (light, short, and fine) to terminal (dark, long, and coarse) because the hormones called *androgens* are activated, which cause hair to change. Androgens can increase the size of the hair follicle, the diameter of the hair fiber (generally called a strand), and the amount of time it spends in its active, growing stage.

Our body create, and circulate, androgens normally during puberty. The androgens also produce a healthy sex drive, called *libido*. All women secrete androgens from their ovaries and adrenal glands, but fat cells and muscle cells can manufacture androgens, too. If you have added significant fat or muscle to your body, you may see an increase in darker, coarser hair—your terminal hair, which, can cause hirsutism due to increased hormone production.

You may have heard of androgens referred to as male sex hormones. Men typically have much higher levels than women. Similarly, all men secrete small amounts of estrogen, which balances out their sex drives, and masculine traits. (Otherwise, they would be covered with dark, coarse hair and resemble primitive man—and their sex drive would be unmanageable!)

Men have more areas on their body—in their skin to be exact—that are sensitive to androgens than women. That is why so many more of their fine, vellus hairs turn into hair that is coarser, longer, and more visible than hair on women's bodies. In fact, it is considered culturally attractive, masculine, and sexy for men to bear hair. A sad change in our culture, however, seems to be a reduced tolerance for men with terminal hair on their back or other parts.

Several places on our body are not androgen dependent, for instance, our hands, feet, eyebrows, and eyelashes. And there is no direct correlation between the normal amount of androgens circulating in our body and our terminal hair's length or rate of growth. Androgen levels, like hair, are controlled by genetics. So for certain people, one level of androgens circulating in their body at a specific developmental stage is normal, and for another group it is different. For instance, there is no difference in the levels of testosterone between Asians and Caucasians, yet the difference in hair quantity between these two groups is the greatest.

Androgen levels change and elevate as our body develop, in puberty, early adolescence, late adolescence, pregnancy, and menopause. These elevated levels occur at different stages of development for males, too. Depending on their genetic makeup, males have different levels of terminal hair, without any correlation to specific androgen levels or their masculinity. For men, frontal balding is related to their androgen levels. You see it starting in the front, which is the same hormonal mechanism women experience with alopecia (scalp hair loss). However, because actual hormone levels vary and are not a one-to-one correlation with hair growth or loss, you cannot infer that a balding man or a man without a lot of hair has any different libido than other men; that is simply a myth.

It is *not* normal for vellus hair on prepubescent girls to change into terminal hair. There have been stories in the medical press and the media about early puberty levels becoming more and more common. Although this may be true, girls with terminal hairs should not be written off by a doctor as entering early puberty. If this happens, insist that the doctor refer your daughter to an endocrinologist if you need a referral, or visit one on your own that specializes in hirsutism. Puberty comes with other indicators besides terminal hair growth and the start date is usually genetic. In addition, some of the terminal hair might be growing in areas where it would not in "normal" conditions. Therefore, if your daughter, sister, or relative has terminal hairs before the age of ten or eleven, or whatever is normal in your family, this might indicate an issue affecting her endocrine system.

Once a woman enters puberty, terminal hair continues to grow gradually and depending on the life of a particular hair. The growth then switches to hair loss after menopause because the ovaries no longer produce androgens. So, yes, your pubic hair will start to lose pigment and fall out, along with other hair. The irony is that you may fret about having hair now only to mourn it when it is gone!

You will also notice more terminal hair during pregnancy. One of the effects of the many hormonal changes is that the line of hair from your belly button to your pubic hair darkens, thickens, and becomes more noticeable, as does the hair on your areolas. You may have more terminal hair in other areas as well. It is strange how discussing this hair growth is omitted from much of the information provided to pregnant women, especially when it can be difficult to deal with, along with all the body's other challenges.

Extra hair during pregnancy and in the postpartum stage does not mean you are hirsute. Like pregnancy itself, your body returns mostly to its pre-pregnant state eventually. It is just another change with which to expect and cope with during pregnancy and during the intense period after the birth of your child.

If your hair growth does not return to prepregnancy levels after your period returns to normal or you are finished nursing, then you may want to consider seeing an endocrinologist. In the meantime, try to avoid removing the hair and possibly aggravating the hair follicle. Remind yourself that the hair will disappear eventually. If you are self-conscious in front of your partner, try sharing your fears with him or her and perhaps you will find some empathy and reassurance. If you can't, bring up your anxiety about the hair growth with your midwife, prenatal exercise class instructor, or a support group. And of course, swapping stories and fears with other pregnant or recently pregnant women is the best treatment of them all, usually good for a few laughs and some relief.

Skin Interactions

I'm losing the hair on my head as I grow older. But now it is coming out my nose! —B.M.

It is actually our skin's reaction to androgens that causes our hair to change or grow. The pattern with which our skin interacts with androgens is determined during the embryonic stage, so there is not a lot you can do about it now.

Here's how it works: An enzyme called *5-alpha-reductase* reacts with the skin. The enzyme's activity (called metabolism) produces the androgens dihydrotestosterone from the bloodstream and circulating testosterone. Dihydrotestosterone binds to the skin, or more specifically, the *pilosebaceous unit*, which induces the hair follicle to produce terminal hair instead of vellus hair. The pilosebaceous unit is made up of a hair shaft, a hair follicle, and a sebaceous gland. The enzyme's activity and the skin's reactivity to dihydrotestosterone are considered genetically based, which is why you see a range of hair growth among different groups of people.

Hair loss and baldness are related to increased hair growth because they stem from the same chemical reactions in our skin. This is why you may see some people with thinning hair on their head, but lots of hair on other parts of their body, especially as they age. Acne is also related, and it is not uncommon to find acne with hirsutism, especially acne occurring well past adolescence.

The medical condition alopecia, which seems to be the opposite of hirsutism because one *loses* hair in body areas sensitive to androgens, is actually related to hirsutism. With certain disorders, one woman may exhibit hirsutism, whereas another has alopecia. These disorders fall under the category of *hyperandrogenism*, which is an overproduction of the hormone androgen. Women in their childbearing years with hyperandrogenism usually have symptoms of menstrual or ovarian dysfunction as well. Hyperandrogenism can be very dangerous and is a precursor to heart disease or diabetes.

Terminal Hair: Dark, Coarse Hair

When a woman's skin and vellus hairs are exposed to increased androgen activity during puberty, pregnancy, different parts of the menstrual cycle, weight or muscle gain, or a myriad of other conditions, hair that used to be fine and light becomes coarser and darker. Terminal hair examples include:

- Pubic hair and hair that extends up the torso (above the belly button or between the breasts)
- Underarm hair (also called axillary hair)
- Leg hair
- Coarse strands of hair around the nipple (also called axillary hair)
- Upper lip hair (these become darker, but not usually coarser)

Unwanted Hair and Hirsutism

Terminal hair in these areas is perfectly normal and common, and indicates that your body is developing properly—that you are becoming a woman and will soon be able to do what only women can, which is to create and nourish life. This is so common, in fact, that comedian Joy Behar, in one of her stand-up routines, exclaimed in her Brooklyn accent: "So, what's with that strand of hair on the breast; you know, that 'singular sensation'—how many of you have this?" The audience is silent. No hands go up. Behar then says, "Oh, great. So it's just me!" The women in the audience roar with laughter, confirming that Behar is definitely not alone!

When women begin to notice terminal hair around puberty, they can aggravate hair growth by plucking out the hair with fingers, tweezers, wax, sugaring, threading, stringing, or electronic devices. If you are in this category, as disconcerting or shocking as the hair is, try to refrain from plucking it out and speak to a parent about some of the alternatives in this book.

TALKING TO YOUR ADOLESCENT GIRL

> *The first time I shaved I had to beg my mom to let me. I sliced my legs all to hell.* —L.J.

L.J.'s mother knew she would be shaving, but there are countless stories of preteens and young teens buying or using their big sister's hair removal products and hurting themselves like L.J., or removing hair that then grows in much darker. Common places preteens and young teens remove their hair are on the forearms and face.

Removing hair is a rite of passage made more urgent by cultural influences. If you are a parent of a preteen or young teen, be sure to discuss hair and its possible removal with your daughter when she begins to enter puberty. Don't wait for all her terminal hair to grow in or for her breasts to develop. Bring up the subject of unwanted hair yourself and offer possible solutions, regardless if your teen is not ready to open up. Even if you have tried to prepare her for puberty, nothing you say can keep her from comparing herself to other teenagers and women. This includes friends and family as well as touched-up women in the media. Comparing oneself and feeling self-conscious are part of adolescence and identity formation. The important thing is for her to find positive and attainable comparisons.

Unwanted Hair and Hirsutism

As a parent, you can also take this time to develop your daughter's media literacy and cultural awareness. If she doesn't live in an area with women who look like her, take a trip overseas or to a city with a large ethnic population like your own, watch some foreign videos or Link TV (currently available on satellite and over the Internet).

You might also show your daughter one of the hairs you have hated or tried to pluck out, as it is likely genetic. Be prepared for her to disparage you as she does herself. Although her comments may feel insulting, use them to start a dialogue about hair. And most importantly, only talk positively or not at all about hair. When you speak about your hair and other women's hair as normal parts of being human, she will learn that message. When you criticize yourself or others, she will be experiencing some of the most negative role modeling possible.

The methods included in the table on the following page are also good to use if your daughter has a prominent nose or is Asian and may be struggling with the shape of her eyes. Plastic surgery has taken a foothold among adolescents, especially in certain regions and populations of the country. The same cultural forces at play for unwanted hair are in play for much of a woman's body; and while she may scare herself removing unwanted hair improperly, plastic surgery could have an even more devastating long-term effect.

Unwanted Hair and Hirsutism

Table 1. How to Help an Adolescent Girl Develop Healthy Attitudes about Hair

1. First, find out when it is the norm for girls in her school to shave and watch for the transformation of her vellus hair into terminal hair.	• Talk to her about her opinions and wishes for hair removal. • Tell her about your experiences and feelings and the positive lessons you have learned. • Show her and talk to her about your hair, or if she has an aunt around with more similarities to her than you do, set the stage for those conversations.
2. Provide opportunities for her to see young women (real or images) who have similar origins and hair or body types. Create a dialogue around what she sees.	• Travel to a city with neighborhoods of similar-origin people. • Rent movies. • Watch Link TV, foreign broadcasts, or other television shows that portray real women from around the world both in news and entertainment. • Travel out of the country. • Find young-adult books that tackle the subject, both fiction and nonfiction. A classic nonfiction book is *Changing Bodies, Changing Lives* (Bell 1998). A recently published book is *Body Drama* (Redd 2008). • Steer her away from mainstream media.
3. Develop her media literacy and cultural awareness. The Web site www.jeankilbourne.com is a good place to start. Or if you don't have Internet access, the library might carry or could order videos and books for you.	
4. Be vigilant about your own attitudes toward hair and what you communicate to her.	
5. Talk to her about hair removal: what works, what doesn't, and what you two can agree on. Then help her make it happen.	

CHAPTER 3

HIRSUTISM: TOO MUCH HAIR

There are many ranges of normal hair growth; no one's family background is abnormally hairy, they just have an amount of hair common for their ethnic type. For example, dark-haired, dark-skinned women with Mediterranean or Middle Eastern backgrounds have more hair on their body than Native American, Asian, or blond, light-skinned northern European women.

Maybe you don't feel normal if your social circle looks different than you, or if you spend a lot of time reading fashion magazines or watching music videos. You cannot change these genetic traits any more than you can change genetic heart disease. It is actually our skin color, hair color, and hair texture that distinguish our racial traits more than does any other feature.

The United States and some other countries have abnormal beauty standards that no women can ever meet, no matter what our origins. Talk to a professional model, and she will tell you the same thing. She may be presented as the ideal woman, but she likely also feels pressure to reach an impossible ideal. Being hairless is a beauty standard that is not only impossible, it is not normal. You are not alone if you are having serious difficulty coping with your body's healthy hair growth. At least 10 to 15 percent of women in the United States share your angst, and the majority of women struggle with accepting hair on some of their body.

Hirsutism may make your struggle even harder. Hirsutism, or abnormal excessive hair growth, often contributes significantly to lower self-esteem and a negative body image. Hirsutism can, and often does, affect one's self-perception and confidence. For many women it is psychologically painful. Some women with hirsutism limit their social interaction and activities. Some develop a habit of holding their hands to their faces while speaking or may feel embarrassed about entering into an intimate relationship. Women with hirsutism can become depressed and isolated. The good news is that both hirsutism and depression are treatable. The treatment for most types of hirsutism actually stops the excessive hair growth.

Hirsutism can rob women of an enjoyable quality of life and self-esteem, and it is a very serious condition that warrants treatment. This is not to say that your normal hair growth can't cause you to feel self-conscious, anxious, or unhappy. Although, in no circumstance does hair growth indicate you are losing your femininity. Helping women cope with unwanted hair is the purpose of this book, but it is not a *condition* that can be treated like hirsutism.

TYPES OF HAIR GROWTH THAT QUALIFY AS HIRSUTISM

As mentioned earlier, levels of hair growth are genetic. Hirsutism is the growth of terminal hair in places one normally has it, only in excessive amounts, or in places typically grown on males. Remember that terminal hair is larger and darker than vellus hairs, so it is particularly more noticeable as it grows. You had hair there all the time, it just wasn't noticeable.

Characteristics of hirsutism include:

- The appearance of pubic or other terminal hair before age eight (if you have a daughter in this category, you should have her checked by a pediatric endocrinologist to avoid future hirsutism)
- The sudden appearance of terminal hair within a short period of time, such as within a few months or a year (this is common as women reach their early thirties)
- The need to shave twice a day
- Only one area of your body where hair growth is excessive, referred to as *focal hirsutism*

If you experience sudden and rapid development of hirsutism, it could indicate another medical problem or disease. Consult an endocrinologist immediately.

WHAT IS HIRSUTISM?

Hirsutism occurs when a woman's hair follicles that would normally produce pale, fine vellus hairs have switched to producing darker, coarser terminal hairs in areas of the body that are sensitive to the hormone androgen. In women with hirsutism, androgen-sensitive areas include (see figure 3, page 43):

- Face, commonly around the chin or as an extension of the hairline
- Thick body hair on the torso (or abdomen), often an extension of the pubic hairline

Unwanted Hair and Hirsutism

- Chest
- Areola (area around the nipples)
- Lower back
- Buttocks
- Inner thigh
- External genitalia

Of course, every woman has terminal hair in most or all of these areas. Hirsutism describes an excess of what is normal for your ethnic group (the stereotype about women growing hairs on their chins as they age isn't a stereotype for no reason!). Hirsutism is not the same as healthy, normal growth that you may *think* is excessive and therefore abnormal, but in actuality is normal.

You need not have excessive hair growth to be considered hirsute; however, hirsutism is diagnosed by observing significant excessive hair growth in several of these areas. More recently, the medical community has recognized focal hirsutism.

Generally, hirsutism starts around puberty and progresses slowly over many years. This is also the progression of hirsutism associated with polycystic ovarian syndrome, or PCOS (see chapter 5 for a detailed discussion). However, if it comes on in your middle or older years, it could indicate an adrenal (glands near one's kidney) or ovarian tumor, as these tumors produce androgen hormones that then cause hirsutism. Rapidly progressing severe hirsutism at any age could indicate a dangerous tumor.

Because many of the disorders associated with hirsutism are genetic, including PCOS and congenital adrenal hyperplasia, or CAH (see chapter 4), hirsutism has been mistakenly considered genetic. But it is the disease or condition that is genetic, not necessarily hirsutism itself, and there are many causes of hirsutism, which are discussed later on in this chapter.

Hirsutism not associated with any particular disease or condition, called *idiopathic hirsutism*, runs in families. About 20 percent of women fall into this category. Idiopathic hirsutism is not a real condition, but is a term for hirsutism that doctors have not been able to associate with any disease or condition. So far no gene has been connected to it, and as scientists learn more, it is possible they will find a correlation. What is known to be genetic, however, is how one's skin reacts to testosterone and thus how vellus hair changes to terminal hair.

Unwanted Hair and Hirsutism

So how is it that some hair follicles remain vellus and some turn dark, coarse, longer, and more noticeable? As mentioned, your hair is developmentally and genetically predisposed to turn terminal during puberty, late adolescence, pregnancy, and menopause. However, if your pilosebaceous unit—the glands and hair follicles in your skin—is exposed to androgens for other reasons (e.g., disease, stress, or diet), the vellus hair could also change to terminal hair. It is wholly dependent on your skin reacting to 5-alpha-reductose activity that causes the change. In other words, your hair might change at one level of androgens whereas your best friend's does not.

For some women, the androgen reaction in their skin doesn't lead to hirsutism; instead they get acne, seborrhea, alopecia, or a combination of two of these conditions. For some women, the androgen effects on their skin turns the terminal hair on their scalp into vellus hair, yet their vellus hair turns terminal in other places (akin to bald men with beards). *Seborrhea* is a treatable red, scaly, itchy rash most commonly seen on the scalp, face, and middle of the chest. Other areas, such as the navel, buttocks, skin folds under the arms, axillary regions (around the underarm, including the lymph nodes), breasts, and groin, may also be affected. In all cases, the androgens reacting with your skin causes the conditions.

Certain levels of androgens trigger this conversion for women, although a certain androgen level does not necessarily correlate to hirsutism (or at least not one that scientists have found). In addition, it is still unclear which factors must be present in the skin to trigger the conversion. Mild hirsutism, in particular, does not indicate abnormally high androgen levels, and because androgen levels differ among ethnic groups, there is no standard for which levels relate to varying degrees of hirsutism. That being said, if androgen levels are double or even higher than the normal range for women at a particular life stage, then the majority will experience hirsutism, acne, seborrhea, or alopecia.

One thing is clear: high androgen levels, also known as hyperandrogenemia, indicate the presence of certain medical conditions such as a tumor. Because moderate to severe hirsutism is usually an indicator of androgen production, endocrinologists will also be on the lookout for other diseases associated with hyperandrogenemia (sometimes referred to as *hyperandrogenic syndrome*) while diagnosing hirsutism.

If you have been diagnosed with hirsutism, there can be many causes and therefore different treatments. Blood tests are used to help determine the cause and treatment.

WHAT IS HYPERTRICHOSIS?

If you have excessive terminal hair in parts of your body other than those listed previously for hirsutism, it is called *hypertrichosis*. The difference between hirsutism and hypertrichosis is that hypertrichosis is excess terminal hair growth in areas of the body that are not sensitive to androgens. These androgen-insensitive areas include the forehead, forearms, toes, and tops of the hands. Hypertrichosis is associated with metabolic disorders such as porphyry and hyperthyroidism, reactions to medications or chemicals, anorexia nervosa, and cancer. There is no specific known cause. Hypertrichosis that is associated to a specific area is called *localized hypertrichosis*.

Porphyria is a group of at least eight related disorders where one's body accumulates *porphyrin precursors*, which are normal body chemicals. The body normally does not accumulate them. Precisely which of these chemicals builds up depends on the type of porphyria. The symptoms arise mostly from effects on the nervous system or the skin, thus the manifestation of excess hair. The disorders are named after the Greek word *porphyrus*, meaning "purple," because the urine of some porphyria patients may be reddish in color due to the presence of excess porphyrins. For more information, contact the American Porphyria Foundation.

Anorexia nervosa is an eating disorder that can lead to death if it is not treated; it harms your body in often irreversible ways. Anorexia interferes with many of your body's functions, including its ability to make and regulate hormones. Anorexics usually have excess hair called lanugo all over their body, not just in the androgen-sensitive areas, to insulate and keep their bodies warm as they lose their fat and muscle. If you have it or see increased hair growth on your daughter or son and suspect anorexia, seek help immediately.

Hyperthyroidism has many symptoms other than hair growth, which is rare, that go hand-in-hand, such as menstrual irregularities. It can be a serious and dangerous disease, and when associated with hypertrichosis, it could indicate a tumor.

Exposure to heavy metals such as hexachlorobenzene can also cause hypertrichosis. Medications that can cause hypertrichosis, include the following:

Unwanted Hair and Hirsutism

- Phenytoin (usually orally administered)
- Diazoxide
- Minoxidil
- Glucocorticoids
- Cyclosporine (also spelled ciclosporin)
- Penicillamine
- Acetazolamide
- Interferon

These are not the brand names, so check for the active ingredients of the medication to determine if you are taking these. Doctors are not always aware of medications' side effects, or consider them to be worth the risk. If you are experiencing unwanted hair growth, contact your doctor immediately and discuss the alternatives, risks, and benefits. See the list of medications in appendix B and the side effects listed on page 161.

You may experience localized hypertrichosis after the following (which are rare):
- A topical application of iodine, psoralens, minoxidil, or steroids
- A minor abrasions or plaster cast
- An infection, vaccination, or long-standing lichen simplex

If addressing the reasons you acquired hypertrichosis does not stop the unwanted hair growth, the only treatment to date is hair removal. As with hirsutism, some hair removal methods may aggravate and stimulate hair growth, or are ineffective if your body has developed hypertrichosis for one of the previously listed causes. A dermatologist can help you address the associated causes and removal. For a list of dermatologists and their specialties, contact the American Academy of Dermatology (AAD) at www.aad.org.

DIAGNOSING HIRSUTISM

It is really no wonder that hirsutism has been difficult to diagnose, considering the different types of hair growth and the varying causes and manifestations.

The first medical description differentiating hirsutism from normal hair growth appeared in 1961 by two doctors doing anthropological research. Drs. D. M. Ferriman and J. D. Gallwey measured women's hair growth to set a benchmark for what determined "normal" hair growth. This research was used to discern whether their patients were experiencing hirsutism. The doctors drew a chart of women's hair growth, now called the Ferriman-Gallwey

Index, or FG scale (figure 3). This scale is the most widely used to assess hirsutism. It evaluates the degree of hair growth in eleven areas of the body, with scores from 0 (no terminal hair) to 4 (the highest) for each body part. It does not include underarm or pubic hair. The total score is determined by adding the scores from the eleven areas. The total score possible is 44. The higher the score, the more severe the hirsutism. Using this scale, hirsutism is diagnosed with a score of 8 or greater. A typical score for someone with hirsutism is between 8 and 29, with an average score of 15.

Figure 3. Modified Ferriman-Gallwey Index

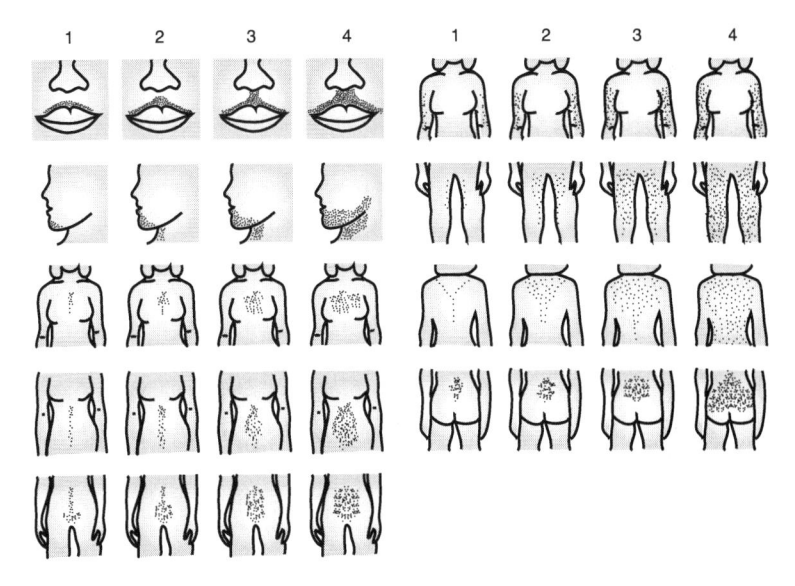

Illustration by Kellie Frissell, www.kfdp.com

The scale has been the standard-bearer for diagnosing hirsutism since it was first developed. This is unfortunate for many women. If the scale is not used properly, a doctor may not suspect a hormonal imbalance and therefore take the proper steps to evaluate the patient's hormone levels. Also, doctors have determined that the FG scale is not accurate for all women because the original study only included women descended from northern Europe and

Unwanted Hair and Hirsutism

Africa. Therefore, if you are not from one of these groups, or you have a mixed background, your "normal" isn't the same. The Endocrine Society uses an example of Asian women, who usually score low on the scale. Although this does not mean that an Asian patient is not hirsute because a low score could be a high indicator for her. In other words, a patient may not appear to be hirsute according to the FG scale, but she should still be diagnosed with hirsutism.

In an effort to correct the scoring, experts have created normative scores for women from Turkish and Thai heritages. For women with Turkish roots, a score up to 11 instead of 8 is normal, and for women with Thai roots, up to 3 is normal. These scores are not widely used in the medical literature, so if you are descended from Turkey or Thailand or the surrounding regions, make sure your endocrinologist is using the correct "normal" baseline score.

Another limitation of the FG scale is that it does not include two common excess growth areas, such as sideburn hair and extragenital hair, which could lead to a misdiagnosis if the doctor primarily uses the scale.

The FG scale also does not measure focal hirsutism. Because each area on the chart is added separately and these totals are then added together, one high area may not raise the total score enough to indicate hirsutism. Therefore, even if you have hirsutism in one area and not in others, you won't show up on the scale as being hirsute.

Today, trained doctors can use a modified FG scale, with its limitations, to help diagnose hirsutism. The FG scale is commonly used to begin diagnosis and to monitor one's progress during treatment, setting a baseline for body parts it does measure.

A trained doctor considers a patient's terminal hair growth in androgen-sensitive areas and takes a history of the growth, a history of her menstrual cycle, and a medication history. Indicators of possible androgen overproduction, such as hirsutism, should alert the doctor to test for hyperandrogenemia, PCOS, a tumor, or other conditions and diseases of the endocrine system. One method is to test the blood for elevated plasma total testosterone levels *after* your body has been resting, which is called an early morning test. Of course, this does not work if you work the night shift or stay up late studying or partying, so be sure to discuss your schedule with your doctor.

The Endocrine Society does not recommend testing for testosterone levels if you have mild hirsutism, which means you won't have to undergo needless tests, but it does recommend hormonal therapy as an option. This is because you are still hirsute even though your androgen levels may appear "normal." The society notes, however, that if the accuracy of androgen tests improve, then administering them may be advisable for more women.

Some medications that cause hirsutism are not detected in blood tests, so the doctor must take an oral history or review your medical charts to determine if you are taking medication now or in the past that is causing the hirsutism. These include anabolic and androgenic steroids, administered to treat endometriosis and sexual dysfunction, or taken by athletes.

If you are an athlete, you may already know about all the side effects of steroids. Hirsutism is just one of them. Your doctor takes confidentiality oaths; therefore if you are taking steroids, be honest with him or her about it. This way you can be evaluated for hirsutism as well as other side effects, such as lactation (producing milk) and depression.

Parents concerned about their athlete-daughter's (including dancers) hair and/or muscle growth, and possible menstrual irregularity, should not discount steroid use. Many people, particularly young adults, take steroids without knowing the side effects. She may not know that performance-enhancing drinks or pills could be powerful drugs. Ask her whether she is trying anything to enhance her performance, such as a drink or a vitamin. If you are concerned, take her to an endocrinologist, who can test her for steroid use if she is wittingly or unwittingly ingesting a steroid.

One medication that increases plasma testosterone levels and shows up during a test, is valproic acid, an anticonvulsant for neurological disorders. If you are taking this drug, talk to your doctor about alternatives or hirsutism treatment that won't interfere with your neurological condition.

For moderate to severe hirsutism, the Endocrine Society recommends testing for elevated androgen levels across the board. It also recommends the test for minor or focal hirsutism and any of the following conditions, to rule out a tumor, PCOS, or another disease (very rare):

- Menstrual irregularity
- Infertility
- Obesity around your midsection
- Acanthosis nigricans (rough, dark skin in the neck folds, nape of the neck, groin, and armpits)

Unwanted Hair and Hirsutism

- Rapidly progressing hair growth
- Enlarged clitoris

After the initial plasma total testosterone test, if the levels are normal but other risk factors are present, or if hirsutism worsens even after hormone therapy, the Endocrine Society recommends patients be tested for total and free testosterone in a qualified laboratory.

If any of the tests find elevated testosterone levels, the next step the Endocrine Society recommends is to rule out the following:
- Pregnancy—with a pregnancy test
- Ovarian tumor or PCOS— with a pelvic ultrasound
- Hyperprolacinemia—by measuring prolactin levels
- Congenital adrenal hyperplasia—by testing for follicular phase levels of 17-hydorxyprogesterone
- Thyroid disorders
- Cushing's syndrome

CONSULTING A DOCTOR

If you suspect you have hirsutism and want to learn more about treatment options, consult an endocrinologist who specializes in hirsutism. An endocrinologist is a medical doctor specially trained in the endocrine system, who diagnoses and treats people with hormonal imbalances.

The endocrine system is considered one of our most important regulatory systems. It is made up of glands, cells, and tissues. The glands make and release hormones into the blood, which travel to tissues and organs throughout the body. The endocrine system regulates the amount of hormones produced and released in our bodies and controls our entire cycle of life, including growth, sleep, sexual development (and terminal hair growth), feelings of hunger and satiation, and the way our body uses food as fuel.

Thus, an endocrinologist diagnoses and treats people with hormonal imbalances by attempting to restore balance. There are many hereditary and severe endocrine disorders, and modern medicine has done wonders to prevent death, birth defects, and disabilities. However, with the increasing rates of type 2 diabetes and PCOS, an endocrinologist can only help so much and patients must also make changes to improve their lives. Alternatively, a patient's stress, diet, sleep patterns, and other factors can cause a hormonal imbalance and an endocrinologist may not be looking for these factors. Environmental causes and medications also have been implicated with endocrine disorders.

Finding a Trained Doctor

You need to see an endocrinologist to receive medical treatment for hirsutism or to rule out any underlying disease or disorder that includes hirsutism as a symptom. A primary care doctor may be able to assess whether you have hirsutism, although he or she may refer you to an endocrinologist for further diagnosis if your seem hormones out of balance. If your doctor believes you do have hirsutism and does not refer you, or she doesn't ask the questions discussed previously, ask for further diagnosis. Also ask for a referral to an endocrinologist who specializes in hirsutism. Ensure you receive the proper attention by using effective language with your primary care doctor or endocrinologist. Try this phrase when speaking to a doctor: "Please rule out a serious underlying disease that may be causing my excessive hair growth."

If you do not have health-care insurance, you can still contact an endocrinologist who specializes in hirsutism and ask about the rates for uninsured patients. Depending on your condition, you may be eligible for Medicaid. All states in the United States offer government health insurance assistance for children under the age of eighteen. Explore these options and do not wait until a potentially dangerous hormonal imbalance occurs. A women's health center or local government health and human services agency can help you apply for government aid or provide reduced-cost care.

Hormonal imbalances are usually correctable or manageable; however, many endocrinologists do not take the condition of unwanted hair seriously in the absence of a hormonal imbalance. Also, many endocrinologists have only an academic "interest" in hirsutism and do not look for possible hormonal imbalances, recommend treatment, or even try to understand the emotional stress it causes. Some even send patients away with vague or inappropriate instructions on how to remove hair and minimize suffering.

Doctors may cite racial or familial genes as a cause of your hirsutism. This is incorrect and demonstrates the doctor's lack of education regarding hirsutism. If your endocrinologist diagnoses you with genetic hirsutism, consult another doctor. The only possible genetic factor is you have a hereditary disease or disorder that causes hirsutism, thus requiring proper diagnosis and treatment. Even idiopathic hirsutism, associated with genetics, can be treated.

If you have been given inaccurate or unhelpful information or have felt "shooed away" by a doctor when asking for help, you are not alone! Many women who have had these experiences end up self-treating, which can do more damage and, in the long run, aggravate hirsutism. It is also likely that you may have encountered a doctor who uses the FG scale as the primary diagnosis tool and does not understand its limitations, and misdiagnoses you.

Ironically, many women uncover a potential hormonal problem during a visit with an electrologist. A trained electrologist may also recognize the symptoms of hirsutism and instruct his or her client to see an endocrinologist.

Fortunately, hirsutism has recently sparked the interest of some in the medical community, including pediatricians. Nevertheless, even medical associations studying hirsutism, such as the Endocrine Society—which produced the definitive guide for endocrinologists evaluating and treating hirsutism among premenopausal women—can have poor information for the actual women suffering from hirsutism or unwanted hair.

Don't give up. If you feel that your concerns are not being met, find another endocrinologist. For a referral to an endocrinologist or other trained specialist, contact one or more of the following:

- The American Electrology Association (www.electrology.com) has a list of caring, knowledgeable endocrinologists. Choose from the menu of physician referrals.
- The American Association of Clinical Endocrinologists (www.aace.com) has a physician referral service under "resources."
- The Hormone Foundation (www.hormone.org) has an easy-to-use physician finder.
- The American Academy of Dermatology (www.aad.org) has a list of dermatologists organized by zip code. You can do a "refined search" for a specialist in your area. Many dermatologists are well versed in hirsutism.

COMMON CAUSES OF HIRSUTISM

As you now realize, the causes of hirsutism are not readily known. Clearly, androgen production and its metabolism are related. Therefore, a treatment that reduces androgen production works for many women, as do lifestyle changes that naturally adjust your body's androgen metabolism and production. In some cases, if you treat the condition, hirsutism disappears as the treatment works.

It is helpful to know what could be causing your hirsutism so that you can treat it properly. You can easily worsen hirsutism accidentally by using hair removal methods that stimulate hair growth. Or if your hirsutism is caused by excess androgens, you will be just wasting time and money on hair removal instead of treating the real cause. Excess androgen production also aggravates hypertrichosis.

The following are the nine most common causes of hirsutism and a few tips on how to avoid them.

Polycystic Ovarian Syndrome

Polycystic ovarian syndrome, or PCOS, is linked to too much androgen production. In recent years it has been studied and diagnosed more frequently. Because this condition is becoming increasingly common among women as obesity rates rise, chapter 5 is entirely devoted to PCOS's causes, symptoms, treatment, and relationship to hirsutism.

Recreational Steroid Use

Recreational steroid use refers to inhaling, injecting, or drinking steroids whether in the form of a drug, "vitamin," or urine from pregnant animals, to build muscle. The popular term is *performance-enhancing drugs*. If you are using them and are already addicted, seek medical help immediately. Your hair growth should return to normal when you stop taking steroids.

Cushing's Syndrome

Cushing's syndrome is rare, and unfortunately 99 percent of the cases are caused by excessive amounts of glucocorticoid, which is used to treat inflammation and immune disorders and diseases, such as asthma, lupus, and arthritis. All patients receiving pharmacologic glucocorticoid treatment develop Cushingoid features if exposed to high doses for one month or more. The signs of hypercortisolism (too much glucocorticoid in one's body) are frequently subtler in pediatric patients than in adults. Usually women with Cushing's syndrome get hirsutism. Since the 1940s, alternative drug treatments have been available.

Unwanted Hair and Hirsutism

Named after Harvey Cushing, who in 1932 was one of the first physicians to report a patient affected with excessive glucocorticoid. When the condition develops naturally, it is usually due to a pituitary tumor; however, it can be associated with an adrenal tumor.

Cushing's syndrome is characterized by central obesity, a moon-shaped face, fat around the neck, and thinning arms and legs. Children are obese and their growth is slowed. It is much more common among women than men by a nine-to-one ratio. If you've taken a glucocorticoid or wonder if you have, consult a specialist who can fully diagnose and treat Cushing's syndrome. For more information, visit www.cushings-help.com.

Drug Side Effects

Many drugs can cause excess androgen secretion and either hirsutism or alopecia (scalp hair loss), in women. These drugs include the following:

- Dilantin (used to control seizures)
- Danazol (used in extreme cases of endometriosis; causes hirsutism in 85 percent of patients)
- Cyclosporine
- L-thyroxine therapy (used in endemic goiter lesions)
- Steroids (used in a variety of drugs, particularly asthma medications and pain relief)
- Oral contraceptives (certain oral contraceptives increase circulating androgen levels, whereas others decrease them)
- Glucocorticoids

If you already have hirsutism, there are some drugs that can increase the level of androgens in your body, thereby aggravating the condition. If you are prescribed one of the medicines in the previous list or one with a side effect of increasing androgen levels, you should discuss these possibilities with your endocrinologist and weigh the benefits of the drugs prescribed against the risks.

As a general rule, whenever you're taking either a prescription or an over-the-counter drug, be sure to ask about common side effects and read the information insert carefully. You can find more in-depth information about how a drug works and possible side effects in the *Physician's Desk Reference*, referred to as the PDR (available at all libraries in the United States, or online at

Unwanted Hair and Hirsutism

www.pdr.net). In Canada, drug information is published in the *Compendium of Pharmaceuticals and Specialties* (CPS), which is available in libraries or online at www.cdnpharm.ca/pubcps.htm.

The terms drug companies use to describe hair growth vary. Be on the look out for the following words or phrases:

- Hirsutism
- Hypertrichosis
- Facial hair
- Excessive hair growth
- Excessive hairiness
- Abnormally excessive growth of hair
- Growth of face, back, chest, or stomach hair
- Increased body hair
- Cushingoid state or Cushing's disease or syndrome
- Virilization

If you are taking steroids for asthma or allergies, these steroids can increase your androgen levels, thus causing or aggravating hirsutism. Discuss alternatives with your allergist and make sure you are taking steps to avoid allergens in your home. See appendix B for a more extensive list of drugs that cause hair growth in women.

Insulin Resistance and Type 2 Diabetes

If your body develops a resistance to insulin, it compensates by secreting more than average amounts of insulin. Insulin works by binding to insulin receptors, which then send signals to your pancreas to regulate its production. If the signal weakens due to the excess insulin, your body does not know to stop production. Continued excess insulin gradually compromises the ability of the pancreas to secrete it, to the extent that the pancreas simply cannot cope and you develop diabetes.

There are two types of diabetes: type 1 diabetes is an autoimmune disease and type 2 diabetes develops as a result of diet and lifestyle, and also has a genetic component. Type 2 is becoming increasingly common in the United States, even among children. For more information, visit the American Diabetes Association at www.diabetes.org, or in Canada, the Canadian Diabetes Association at www.diabetes.ca.

Unwanted Hair and Hirsutism

Excess insulin has a tendency to lay fats cells around the waist and inside the stomach, as well as to cause fat infiltration in the muscles, liver, and even heart. Insulin also turns on the enzymes in the ovaries and adrenal glands that make sex hormones. These resulting excess androgens often cause hirsutism.

Perhaps having hirsutism or the fear of getting it will serve as another motivation to take care of your body, thus curing you of this double-whammy. If your young daughter is obese or gaining too much weight, be on the lookout for hirsutism; she doesn't need another physical problem in this difficult stage of her life.

Although, it has become increasingly difficult for Americans to eat a healthy diet, so it is no easy feat to reduce the risk of developing diabetes. Here are a few ideas that might help:

- Learn to avoid processed foods, the majority of restaurant chains, and sodas or sugary fruit drinks that can become a habit for you.
- Take advantage of a referral to a nutritionist or coach that your health insurance carrier or employer offers.
- Try shopping in local food co-ops, farm stands, farmers' markets, and stores that sell natural foods. Co-ops and natural food stores also usually offer health tips and support.
- Bag your own lunches and snacks and teach your children to cook. It is also more affordable.

Rare Endocrine Disorders

Several rare endocrine disorders can cause your androgen levels to increase to the point where you are considered to have hyperandrogenemia. These disorders are usually accompanied by hirsutism.

Nonclassic congenital adrenal hyperplasia (NCAH) is the most common of these. It is a family of inherited disorders affecting the adrenal glands in severe or mild forms. The severe form, called classical CAH, is usually detected in the newborn period or in early childhood. The milder form, NCAH, may cause symptoms at any time from infancy through adulthood.

CAH is an autosomal recessive genetic disorder. For a child to be born with either form of CAH, both parents must carry a gene for the disorder. Scientists have pinpointed the location of the group of genes that causes the most common forms of CAH to chromosome 6. This particular group of genes contain instructions the adrenal glands (located on top of the kidneys) need to produce an enzyme called *hydroxylase* (21-hydroxylase being the most frequent within this group of enzymes). Without it, the adrenal glands are unable to produce cortisone, a hormone necessary for life.

Fortunately, CAH can be managed with medication, and with adequate care affected individuals go on to live normal lives. DNA testing is available for the diagnosis of CAH and to detect carriers of the gene mutations. It is important to diagnose or rule out CAH because specific treatment is available, which also reverses hirsutism.

- *Hyperandrogenic insulin-resistant acanthosis nigricans* (HAIRAN syndrome) is a disorder that affects from 1 to 5 percent of all women who secrete too much androgen.
- *Ovarian stromal hyperthecosis* is a disorder in which ovarian cells secrete large amounts of testosterone and DHT.
- *Hyperprolactinemia* is a rare condition of increased prolactin levels in the body (prolactin is necessary for milk production). It can be due to hypothalamic disease or a pituitary tumor, which are associated with hirsutism. Elevated prolactin levels can be seen in up to 20 percent of patients with PCOS.
- *Acromegaly* is a condition that results when the pituitary gland secretes excessive growth hormone after the end of adolescence. Overproduction before the end of adolescence results in gigantism (growing over seven or eight feet in height). Commonly misdiagnosed, acromegaly results in death from cardiovascular disease or cancer. It progresses slowly, causing disability. Hirsutism is also associated with the disorder in the majority of cases among women.

A pituitary tumor may cause the excessive growth hormone secretion. Acromegaly is usually treatable with medication or surgery.

For more information about these disorders, visit the National Organization of Rare Diseases at www.rarediseases.org.

Unwanted Hair and Hirsutism

Obesity

Fat cells can make androgen just as they can make estrogen, thus causing hirsutism. Obese women are at risk for atherosclerosis and coronary heart disease as well as estrogen-dependent cancers such as breast, endometrial, and ovarian cancers, more so than women with healthier levels of body fat.

A person whose weight is mostly distributed around the upper body and abdomen (with thin legs) has a body type that is associated with insulin resistance, and thus hirsutism.

Some rare endocrine disorders are also more likely to develop with obesity, not only causing hirsutism but also other features of too much testosterone and androgens. Reversing obesity takes a long time and is no easy task. In addition to shedding the pounds, as part of the treatment for hirsutism, you must change your lifestyle. It is awfully hard to increase your activity levels when you are putting on weight. The energy and momentum one needs is physical and mental. Try the tips in the following list to increase physical activity. Exercising also helps to regulate your body's endocrine system and to sleep better.

- Be easy on yourself and take small steps as you begin.
- Do household chores on a regular basis.
- Use a trainer.
- If you need physical therapy, get it, because it will help you start becoming active and exercise without injury.
- Use a support group.

Stress

In response to stressful situations, your adrenal glands release stress hormones that speed up your body. As a result, your heart rate increases and your blood sugar levels rise so that glucose can be diverted to your muscles in case you have to move quickly. This is known as the fight-or-flight response. These hormones are called the catecholamines, which are broken down into epinephrine (adrenaline) and norepinephrine.

However, because your adrenal glands also make androgen, increased stress can increase circulating androgens in your bloodstream, particularly the steroid cortical hormone. Our body needs this hormone to deal with physical and emotional stress and to maintain adequate energy supply and blood sugar levels, although; high amounts of these androgens can cause hirsutism. Great, huh? You are already stressed and now you have unwanted hair to stress about!

Some stressors appear at times of intense pressure, such as losing a loved one, bankruptcy, illness, or being sexually or physically abused. Psychologists have a stress rating system that measures a combination of life events, such as moving, having a child, marriage, and so forth. A combination of factors can cause incredible stress, whether or not they negative or positive stressors.

Other types of stress may be present over long periods of time, leaving you angry or depressed. Stress is not to be taken lightly. If you are experiencing excessive hair growth, your body is likely reacting in other ways as well, or perhaps your emotions make you feel as though you have morphed into someone else. In addition to seeking support from friends, family, or professionals, be sure to regularly sleep, eat healthy meals, and exercise, exercise, exercise, even if it is just walking around the block. Once your body regulates, your hair will, too.

Tumors

Tumors of an ovary or the adrenal cortex are associated with hirsutism. Some tumors can secrete androgens, and they are called androgen-secreting tumors. One symptom of an androgen-secreting tumor is rapidly progressing hirsutism. While rare, some of the tumors can be very dangerous. One type is seen in 0.2 percent of premenopausal women with excess androgen production, and half of these tumors are malignant. Another type is seen in genetic males with female genitalia.

A pituitary tumor found to cause hirsutism afflicts people with Cushing's syndrome. There are other less common tumors found with Cushing's syndrome as well.

Related Symptoms

Cushing's disease, PCOS, anorexia nervosa, hypothyroidism, and other conditions are also accompanied by irregular menstrual cycles or periods, in addition to hirsutism. If you have irregular menstrual cycles or they have ceased altogether too early for menopause, this is an indication of something wrong with your endocrine system. Consult a doctor immediately.

CHAPTER 4

TREATMENTS FOR HIRSUTISM

Your doctor should reassure you that hirsutism has nothing to do with femininity, and encourage you to discuss your concerns and questions openly. Often hirsutism is one characteristic among others associated with men, such as muscle growth, balding, and a deep voice. These traits are caused by hormonal imbalances that can be rectified; it does not mean you will grow a penis and become a man. For example, consider hair growth during pregnancy. You are in fact hairier, yet only women can conceive. Your identity as a woman is much more complex and comes from your internal perspective as much as anything else.

An endocrinologist is not a therapist, however, and he or she focuses on diagnosis and treatment, not so much on your psychic suffering. If you are not satisfied with your doctor's rapport, seek out a psychotherapist who is experienced or willing to understand hirsutism. If you are not satisfied with your doctor's explanations and instructions, seek out another endocrinologist.

Treating hirsutism necessitates finding its biological cause, therefore the entire process can take quite a while and involve a lot of testing. A doctor is systematic and does not jump to conclude idiopathic hirsutism, or that nothing is wrong because he or she doesn't see much hair. Your participation and honesty are important for a proper diagnosis.

You do not want a doctor who uses only the Ferriman-Gallwey scale to diagnose your symptoms. In fact, the Endocrine Society, which has produced the most comprehensive and up-to-date guide for medical doctors to evaluate and treat hirsutism, recommends that doctors do *not* use the FG scale to decide which treatment to use. The primary reason is that the FG scale can't accurately measure a woman's hair growth if she has already been removing it. The medical community is finally comprehending that women who grow up in the United States begin removing their unwanted body hair soon after they hit puberty when they see terminal hair grow. It seems like a no-brainer, but this warning is now appearing in medical literature regarding using the FG scale accurately.

Your doctor definitely should not recommend "cosmetic" hair removal instead of or before providing you with a formal diagnosis and treatment plan. Some medical patient material advises women to try cosmetic hair removal before seeking medical care, as if it is a new idea that they need to tell women about, or that a woman would go through the trouble of seeing a doctor without trying something herself, even if it's a tweezer.

Suggesting cosmetic measures before diagnosis is especially bad advice for girls exhibiting hirsutism or for women with moderate to severe hirsutism because (1) hirsutism likely indicates a serious medical condition and (2) many removal techniques only make the terminal hair growth worse. Girls with terminal hair growth in early puberty should be seen immediately by an experienced doctor.

During a diagnosis, an endocrinologist conducts a series of tests to exclude certain disorders. If no other disorders are found, the diagnosis is idiopathic hirsutism (or a *diagnosis by exclusion*). However, if an underlying cause is found, it will define the treatment recommended by the doctor. In some cases, such as with tumors, you may need to see another type of doctor as well.

Other than doing nothing about your hair growth (which many women choose to do), in its latest treatment guidelines (the most comprehensive to date) the Endocrine Society recommends two types of treatments for hirsutism—cosmetic hair removal or pharmacological (drug or hormone) therapy. Another option is lifestyle changes with or without pharmacological or cosmetic treatment. An endocrinologist focuses on your hormones, however, and is not likely to spend much time discussing your lifestyle.

Your best bet if you are overweight, feel anxious about exercising, have an eating disorder, or want more information on healthy eating is to ask your doctor about complementary treatments or combining hair removal or hormone treatment with nutritional coaching, physical therapy (if you have joint pain or muscle pain), or psychotherapy. Your endocrinologist may not be well versed in these areas, but hopefully is eager to see you engaged in your own well-being. And if not, you can try these other approaches without your endocrinologist's participation.

Unwanted Hair and Hirsutism

COSMETIC HAIR REMOVAL

Hair removal does not treat hirsutism, and cannot be considered a treatment; however, it is a method to cope with hirsutism. The Endocrine Society's recommendations for cosmetic measures do not address the cause of hirsutism, which means despite cosmetic hair removal, your terminal hair will continue to grow. Therefore, if your aim is to stop the excessive hair growth, cosmetic measures do not work.

There is one exception, which is for facial hair growth. The topical prescription cream *eflornithine* can reduce hair growth in some women. (See section on topical skin cream later in the chapter.) If your aim is to remove unwanted hair, only one type of cosmetic hair removal is permanent, and that is electrolysis (discussed in detail in chapter 7).

You may choose to continue your path of removing the hair or doing nothing and letting it grow, opting not to try hormone therapy. You should discuss the ramifications of this choice with your doctor, however. Sometimes mild hirsutism is associated with PCOS and it may be unwise to go too long without hormone treatment.

If you decide not to try hormone therapy at this time, you can also be measured periodically to ensure your hirsutism does not worsen, as there is a possibility that an underlying cause may exist. Also there is a chance that with a doctor's monitoring you will be diagnosed more specifically in the future. For instance, researchers are now testing 5-apha-reductase activity in skin for its relationship to hirsutism.

HORMONE AND PHARMACOLOGICAL TREATMENTS

If you have idiopathic hirsutism, hormone therapy may not work. Although it has been shown to work in many cases, results are not guaranteed. If you decide to try it and it does not work, you can try hair removal methods or do nothing.

Perhaps you want to try pharmacological therapy or your doctor recommends it to treat an underlying cause, which in turn treats the hirsutism. It can take at least six months to demonstrate results since your hair must cycle through its three stages to assess if the treatment is effective. In many cases, hormone therapy improves but does not fully stop hirsutism.

Your doctor should tell you that none of the drugs used to treat hirsutism are approved by the FDA for such use at the time of this book's writing.

However, many of the treatments target the underlying cause, not specifically hirsutism, so treating hirsutism is the secondary outcome. You may have to sign a consent form.

Hormone therapy and pharmacological drugs do not make the excess hair you already have disappear, but they can stop the growth of new hair. Sometimes this therapy will thin the terminal hair, or make the strands a little lighter. However, the reduction in hirsutism lasts only as long as you take the therapy, with occasional positive effects continuing for a short time after you stop.

Pharmacological therapy might have side effects that you'll need to weigh against the problem of hirsutism. Be sure to ask your doctor about all common side effects of the recommended therapy so that you know what to expect.

You can also try combining pharmacological therapy and cosmetic treatment. During therapy, if you cannot wait for the hair to finish its normal cycle and shed, you will need to use another hair removal method that does not stimulate hair growth. Be sure to discuss hair removal methods with your doctor so that both efforts coincide.

The hormone treatment and drugs discussed next in this chapter have been tested specifically to treat hirsutism. Although medical research continues around the world you should only consider these treatments as a basis for your own research and seek the latest information from your endocrinologist. You can try one treatment course to see if it is satisfactory; however, be aware that there may be more aggressive treatments that yield better results. Doctors generally try a minimal level of a drug or treatment with fewer side effects first to see if it is effective, before they try a more aggressive treatment. Your doctor's idea of effectiveness may be different than yours; therefore, be open and honest about your satisfaction level and the risks you are willing to take.

If you have a particular disorder or a rare disease, you will need a specific treatment to counteract those disorders, and in doing so you may stop or reduce your hirsutism. Your doctor will advise you based on your particular biology and disorder. If you have a tumor, you will likely be on a much faster treatment regimen. Because some rare disorders have a poor prognosis, your doctor must diagnose you as soon as possible. Surgery may be indicated.

Chapter 5 is entirely devoted to PCOS because it is so strongly associated with hirsutism. The treatment information in this chapter is also relevant if you are overweight, obese, insulin resistant, or diabetic.

Unwanted Hair and Hirsutism

Pregnancy

If you are trying to conceive, two recommended hormone treatments for hirsutism should not be used. Discuss your interest in conceiving and your goals with your endocrinologist, including your pregnancy history and history of trying to conceive. Depending on the urgency, you may prefer to wait to treat the hirsutism or carefully weigh the side effects of the choices to see if they are worthwhile.

Infertility, however, can be associated with hyperandrogenism and PCOS, so by treating hirsutism with an antiandrogen or undergoing treatment for PCOS now, you may be increasing your likelihood of conceiving in the future. Individual circumstances vary so you will need to consult with your endocrinologist about what treatment is correct for you.

Oral Contraceptives

The Endocrine Society recommends oral contraceptives (OCs) for the majority of women who want to stop hirsutism. New-generation OCs have low-hormone doses and are much different and varied than they were years ago. OC preparations have differing hormones, including weak antiandrogens. When you compare the chemical recipes of today's OC brands with those of thirty years ago, it is like comparing a Commodore 64 (the very first home computer, circa 1980) with the latest laptop computer.

Not only has the estrogen content been substantially reduced, so has the progestin content. The OCs of yesteryear were also all *monophasic*, meaning that the dose did not change over the course of the cycle. In other words, monophasic OC release estrogen and progestin in constant doses. *Triphasic* OCs deliver different doses of hormones over the course of the cycle, designed to minimize side effects. When the progestin is triphased it delivers less hormone, but is equally effective. In essence, you get more "bang for your buck."

Doctors may default to treating your hirsutism with OCs if you are in your childbearing years, assuming you are sexually active or do not want to conceive. Do not let your doctor make inferences about you, your lifestyle, or your interest in conceiving. Make sure you know the treatment choices.

Oral contraception is about four thousand years old. There is a long history of women orally consuming potions and other toxic concoctions to prevent pregnancy. Women in China drank mercury to prevent conception.

Women in India swallowed carrot seeds as a morning-after contraceptive in the 1500s. Backwoods women in northern New Brunswick drank dried beaver testicles brewed in a strong alcoholic solution. And women in Central America still brew a contraceptive tea and drink it periodically during their menstrual cycle. This tea is the basis of modern OC pills, which were developed in the 1930s from the Central American plant barbasco roota. This led to the discovery of steroids, an integral ingredient of today's OCs.

Today's popular combination contraceptives contain a potent, synthetic estrogen called *ethinyl estradiol*, as well as *progestin*. Most progestins are derived from testosterone; however, some progestins, such as *cyproterone acetate* and *drospirenone*, are structurally unrelated to testosterone and interfere with the androgen receptors in your body.

OCs work by suppressing the androgens secreted by your ovaries, thereby reducing free androgen concentrations in your body and slightly reducing androgen secreted by your adrenal glands. This is a simplified description, but in general terms, contraception works on many levels in your endocrine system to block the processes that cause androgen excess and therefore hirsutism.

The Endocrine Society does not recommend one OC over another for treating hirsutism, but suggests avoiding levonorgestrel, the most androgenic progestin, and instead choosing an OC prepared with *norgestimate* or *desogestrel*, or with a progestin-exhibiting antiandrogenic activity such as drospirenone and cyproterone acetate. The society suggests using a contraceptive with low-dose ethinyl estradiol for suppressing ovarian androgens, noting that no studies have been done to verify its effects on hirsutism but that low doses effectively treat acne (also caused by excess androgens).

If you don't smoke and are healthy, it is safe to take a combination OC from the time of your first period (called *menarche*) until menopause. In fact, there are a number of fringe health benefits to being on OCs, known by clinicians as "noncontraceptive benefits." Because contraceptives prevent ovulation, they also help prevent diseases associated with the ovaries, such as ovarian cancer, ovarian cysts, and endometrial cancer.

Unwanted Hair and Hirsutism

In fact, if you have no children, staying on an OC will have the same therapeutic effects on your ovaries as pregnancy and breastfeeding because it will give your ovaries a "break." The following are considered clear, undisputed benefits of OCs, in addition to excellent contraception:

- Reduce the incidence of endometrial and ovarian cancers
- Reduce the likelihood of developing fibrocystic breast condition
- Reduce the likelihood of developing ovarian cysts
- Reduce the chance of developing iron deficiency anemia due to less menstrual blood loss and more regular cycles
- Reduce the severity of menstrual cramps and premenstrual syndrome (PMS)
- Tend to improve androgen-related side effects such as acne or unwanted facial hair
- Improve cholesterol levels depending on the type of OC

Note that progestin derived from testosterone may also cause side effects, called *androgenic side effects* or *nuisance effects*, including weight gain, acne, and terminal hair (often on one's face). Older-generation progestins are more likely to cause these side effects. In fact, most women who discontinue using their OCs do so because of the androgenic side effects—and that's understandable! If you are one of these women discuss the new generation OCs and their side effects with your doctor to see which one may work for you.

An endocrinologist knows how to prescribe the correct OC, although a general practitioner or ob/gyn might not be aware of the side effects or may not consider them important. If these symptoms occur after you have started an OC program, consult with your doctor or endocrinologist about switching to a different OC.

See tables 2 and 3 for a complete list of side effects. For more information about oral contraceptives, visit the Planned Parenthood Web site at www.plannedparenthood.org. To find out which OCs are best for you, see Appendix C and consult your doctor.

Unwanted Hair and Hirsutism

Table 2. Estrogen-Related Side Effects of Oral Contraceptives

Caused by Too Much Estrogen	Caused by Too Little Estrogen
splotchy face	bleeding/spotting days 1 to 9
chronic nasal congestion	continuous bleeding/spotting
flu symptoms	flow decrease
hay fever/allergies	pelvic relaxation symptoms
urinary tract infections	vaginitis atrophic
bloating*	
dizziness*	
edema (water retention)*	
headaches*	
irritability*	
leg cramps*	
nausea/vomiting*	
visual changes*	
weight gain*	
cervical changes	
breast cysts	
dysmenorrhea (painful periods)	
heavy flow and clotting	
increase in breast size	
excessive vaginal discharge	
uterine enlargement	
uterine fibroid growth	
capillary fragility	
blood clots and related disorders	
spidery veins on the chest area	

*These are also PMS-related symptoms.
Source: R. P. Dickey, M.D., Managing Contraceptive Pill Patients, *12th edition, Essential Medical Information Systems, 2004*

Unwanted Hair and Hirsutism

Table 3. Progestin-Related Side Effects of Oral Contraceptives

Caused by Too Much Progestin	Caused by Too Little Progestin
appetite increase	bleeding/spotting days 10 to 21
depression	delayed withdrawal bleeding
fatigue	dysmenorrhea
hypoglycemia symptoms	heavy flow and clots
weight gain	bloating*
hypertension	dizziness*
leg veins dilated	edema*
cervicitis	headache*
flow length decrease	irritability*
yeast infections	leg cramps*
acne**	nausea/vomiting*
jaundice**	visual changes*
hirsutism**	weight gain*
libido increase**	amenorrhea
libido decrease	
oily skin and scalp**	
rash and pruritis**	
edema**	

*These are also PMS-related symptoms. ** Due to excess androgen.
Source: R. P. Dickey, M.D., Managing Contraceptive Pill Patients, *12th edition, Essential Medical Information Systems, 2004*

Common Questions about Oral Contraceptives

Q. Exactly how much weight can I expect to gain?

A. The newer OCs on the market are designed to minimize appearance-related side effects, such as weight gain. Nevertheless, the latest studies show that women who do gain weight tend to gain less than three pounds.

Unwanted Hair and Hirsutism

Q. At what age should I stop using an OC?

A. If you're on a low-dose OC you can stay on the pill right up until menopause so long as you're healthy and don't smoke. When you reach fifty, your doctor may decide to pull you off your OC to see if you're in menopause. That means you'll simply not get your period after being off the OC. Or, your doctor can check your follicle stimulating hormone (FSH) levels; if they're high, you're in menopause. At that point, you'll probably need to discuss options such as hormone replacement therapy, natural hormone replacement therapy, or natural menopause.

Q. Can I take an OC if I smoke?

A. Technically, if you're under thirty-five and smoke, you still can take a combination OC, but you're at greater risk for blood clots, which could lead to a stroke. If you're over thirty-five and smoke, you should not take a combination OC, although you may be able to take the progestin-only pill (the "mini-pill"). Be sure to evaluate all other health risks before choosing this option.

Q. What if I want to get pregnant in a few years?

A. OCs do not interfere with future fertility. When you're ready to get pregnant, finish your package and wait for at least one natural period before you try to conceive. Use a backup method of birth control while you're waiting.

Antiandrogen Therapy

Your doctor may recommend an antiandrogen to inhibit androgen receptors in your body—that is, hair follicles. Antiandrogens can reduce hirsutism by 30 to 60 percent and reduce the diameter of hair shafts. They are dose dependent and your doctor may try different doses. Antiandrogens should not be used if you are sexually active without excellent contraception because the hormones can cause fetal *pseudohermaphroditism* (external genitalia of one sex and internal sex organs of the other sex) in males if used during pregnancy. Your doctor should discuss your lifestyle with you and treatment options if you are in your childbearing years. The following are the antiandrogens used to treat hirsutism:

Unwanted Hair and Hirsutism

Spironolactone
Spironolactone works by inhibiting androgen receptors and 5-alpha-reductase activity. The size of the dose also is associated with menstrual irregularity. However, if taken with an oral contraceptive, there is no irregularity. It may cause dizziness early in the treatment and diuresis (you will urinate more frequently). It is not recommended if you are at risk for osteoporosis.

Finasteride
Finasteride also works by inhibiting 5-alpha-reductase activity. The most beneficial dose effectiveness has not been determined at the time of this book's writing. Prolonged use of spironolactone is more effective than finasteride therapy.

Cyproterone Acetate
Cyproterone acetate (CPA) is not available in the United States although it is used worldwide for both hirsutism and acne treatment. CPA has some degree of inhibiting 5-alpha-reductase activity. It suppresses *serum gonadotropin* and androgen levels. It is as beneficial as other antiandrogens in treating hirsutism if combined with ethinyl estradiol as an oral contraceptive.

Drospirenone
Drospirenone is a weak antiandrogen. This progestin is used in several oral contraceptives. In a combination OC, its effectiveness treating hirsutism is similar to an OC with CPA.

Flutamide
Flutamide works by blocking androgen uptake and binding. Data suggest that flutamide is more effective than finasteride. At doses lower than 250 mg, it is not effective for hirsutism. However, because higher doses can cause hepatic toxicity resulting in liver failure or death, its use should be monitored closely.

Antiandrogen Creams
Antiandrogen creams have limited efficacy. Local application of spiro-nolactone seems to have some benefits whereas finasteride has had inconsistent results.

Antiandrogens and Oral Contraceptives
There is indication that adding spironolactone or finasteride to an oral contraception increases the effectiveness of treating hirsutism. The Endocrine Society recommends this treatment for a patient if results are unsatisfactory after at least six months on either an oral contraceptive or an antiandrogen. Regarding using OCs versus antiandrogens, there has been only one test between the two to date, and it tested finasteride. No difference was found between using finasteride and an oral contraceptive containing a low-dose CPA.

Insulin-Lowering Drugs
You may be prescribed *metformin* or *thiazolidinediones* to address insulin resistance or diabetes. These drugs stabilize or reduce androgen production. Hirsutism decreases at about the same rate as it does with an OC, but insulin-lowering drugs are much less effective than taking an antiandrogen. Adding metformin to the flutamide produced no difference in hirsutism. Because the side effects of these drugs are severe, they are not recommended to treat hirsutism alone.

Glucocorticoid Therapy
In women with classic congenital adrenal hyperplasia, or CAH, glucocorticoids are prescribed to suppress adrenal androgens and to maintain normal *adulatory* cycles. As a result, hirsutism is prevented or improved. In non-classic CAH, the glucocorticoids role in treating hirsutism is less effective.

For women with hyperandrogenemia, including those with PCOS, glucocorticoid therapy appears to reduce hirsutism due to its effect on adrenal androgen production (as opposed to ovarian androgen production). At low doses, glucocorticoids reduce adrenal androgen secretion without significantly inhibiting cortical production (which has many side effects, including Cushing's syndrome), but they also do not suppress serum testosterone levels effectively enough to be more than mildly effective in reducing hirsutism. Higher doses of glucocorticoids can be dangerous and even at recommended doses slight overdosing can occur. One benefit is that after glucocorticoid therapy hirsutism remains reduced for some time.

GnRH Agonists
Normally used in fertility treatment, *gonadotropin releasing hormones* (GnRH), such as the follicle stimulating hormone (FSH), are used to kick-start the ovaries. When FSHs are suppressed, the ovary does not make estrogen or androgens. GnRH therapy improves hirsutism among women with ovarian hyperandrogenism. Uncontrolled studies have found that GnRH agonist therapy is as effective as OC therapy, but when GnRH therapy is combined with low-dose estrogen plus progestin it is more effective than an OC therapy alone; in addition there is evidence the hair growth returns more slowly. At present only one study comparing GnRH therapy to antiandrogen therapy and GnRH therapy has proved more effective in treating hirsutism. However, severe estrogen deficiency results with GnRH agonist therapy and women can experience hot flashes and bone loss. Treatment requires injections and estrogen supplements.

Stress Treatment
If you are prescribed a medication to relieve anxiety, depression, or anger, be sure to discuss the side effects with your doctor and to discuss your concerns about hirsutism. An endocrinologist treating you for hirsutism may be more likely to interpret the effects of the medication on your hirsutism than your primary care doctor or psychiatrist.

Psychotherapy, group therapy, counseling, exercise, lifestyle changes, or reducing or adjusting to stressors should all reduce the amount of androgens your body produces, therefore reducing your hirsutism.

Obesity Treatment
Pharmacological treatment is just starting to enter the market. No studies have been done on their ability to reduce hirsutism, but reduction in fat either from medication, lifestyle changes, or surgery will reduce one's androgen production and therefore should reduce hirsutism.

Topical Skin Cream
A topical cream *called eflornithine hydrochloride cream* (13.9 percent) for the face reduces the rate of hair growth for many women. It is an irreversible inhibitor of ornithine decarboxylase, an enzyme necessary for hair growth. Results are noticeable in six to eight weeks. Once the application of the

cream is discontinued, hair returns to pretreatment levels after about eight weeks. The FDA prescription, called *Vaniqa* (no generics available), can be used alone or in conjunction with other therapies. Skin irritation has been reported only with experimental conditions of overuse. Side effects include itching, dry skin, temporary redness, stinging, burning, or tingling.

Vaniqa has about a 60 percent success rate, but if you have hirsutism that affects your face, you may want to give it a try. White women and postmenopausal women have slightly better success rates. It has not been tested on pregnant or breast-feeding women; so as with any chemicals, do not use it in those circumstances.

Common Questions about Vaniqa

Q. How do I use Vaniqa?
A. Vaniqa is rubbed into the surface of your skin, which slows the growth within the hair follicle itself. Over time you do notice that you will not have to remove your hair as often.

Q. How will I know if it is effective?
A. Decide with your doctor an appropriate time to stop the treatment if your hair growth has not slowed after eight weeks.

Q. Does health insurance cover the prescription?
A. In some cases, yes. Study your policy and consult with your doctor. You may have to advocate for it, but since it is so expensive, your efforts should pay off.

Q. How does Vaniqa affect my makeup or sunscreen?
A. It doesn't as long as you wait for the application to dry before you apply any cosmetics to your face.

Q. If I wash my face after applying Vaniqa, will it still work?
A. Probably not as well. It is advised to wait at least four hours before you wash your face or wet it (e.g., swimming) after applying Vaniqa.

Q. Will my hair growth be worse after stopping Vaniqa?
A. Your hair will simply grow as it did before you used Vaniqa: no less, no more. Vaniqa needs to be stopped for an extended period of time before hair growth resumes. If you miss one or two applications, it is not going to make a difference.

Other Treatments
Diet drinks, pills, herbs, and supplements often are not FDA approved. You should discuss any alternative treatments with your endocrinologist to see if there are side effects that could influence hirsutism. As of this book's writing, no treatments other than what is described in this chapter are approved. Be aware of many scams available in stores, through television shopping, and on the Internet.

CHAPTER 5

POLYCYSTIC OVARIAN SYDROME: THE MOST COMMON CAUSE OF HIRSUTISM

Roughly 6 to 10 percent of the general female population suffers from polycystic ovarian syndrome (PCOS), which is also called Stein-Leventhal syndrome (after the two doctors that defined it in 1935) or polycystic ovary disease (PCOD). Although these numbers sound shockingly high, approximately 25 to 33 percent of women in their childbearing years actually have PCOS. Worse, most women don't know they have it and most doctors don't screen for it during regular physicals.

PCOS can start at any time during a woman's reproductive life. Generally, a woman with PCOS will begin to experience menstrual irregularities within three to four years after her menarche (first period). It is uncommon to develop PCOS later in life, although it can happen. What might be more realistic is that a woman developed it during her teen years but it wasn't diagnosed until she was older (and perhaps reading this book!). It also accounts for half of all hormonal disorders affecting female infertility, in addition to causing hirsutism. Women rarely develop PCOS after delivering a baby.

PCOS can afflict girls as young as ten or twelve years old. Girls who experience early puberty (or the appearance of pubic hair and breasts at age seven or eight) have a very high risk of subsequent PCOS, as do girls with childhood obesity.

POSSIBLE SYMPTOMS OF PCOS

Approximately 70 percent of women with PCOS have hirsutism on their face and/or body. Other symptoms include the following:

- Irregular or absent menses (periods)
- Cysts on one's ovaries (often women don't know they have cysts; they may feel pain in general, while walking or running, or during sexual intercourse, and other times they don't; sometimes the cysts dissolve on their own, often causing painful periods, and sometimes they don't and need to be removed by a doctor)

Unwanted Hair and Hirsutism

- High blood pressure
- Acne, particularly if it first appears significantly in adulthood
- Elevated insulin levels, insulin resistance, or diabetes
- Infertility
- Thinning hair on one's scalp (alopecia, see page 33 for more information)
- Weight problems or obesity centered around a woman's midsection (obesity is often associated with PCOS, although women who are thin or who have a healthy weight may also have it)
- Early puberty, or the appearance of pubic hair and breasts at age seven or eight.
- Delayed or absent puberty
- Secondary amenorrhea (normal menstrual cycles become irregular)
- Unexplained fatigue
- Sugar cravings
- Hypoglycemia, or low blood sugar, occurring after or between meals
- Mood swings
- Hot flashes in young women (characterized by heat intolerance and excess sweating)
- Sleep disorders, particularly sleep apnea (reduction in or cessation of breathing while you sleep)
- Recurring miscarriages
- Milk leaking from one's breasts (lactating without having a baby)
- Low blood pressure, noticeable when one stands up suddenly or after exercise
- Rough, dark skin in one's neck folds, nape of the neck, groin, and armpits, known as acanthosis nigricans (sometimes dark coloring only in certain areas of the skin is referred to as hyperpigmentation)

The signs of PCOS range from the subtle, such as irregular periods and excess facial hair, to what is called the *full-house syndrome*. The latter can mean no periods, obesity, hirsutism, diabetes, and cardiovascular disease. A full 5 percent of women in their childbearing age have this severe type.

The early diagnosis and treatment of girls and women is vital. Only through early diagnosis and treatment can a woman avoid experiencing PCOS progress to its more severe, full-house syndrome.

Although not known conclusively, an underlying cause of PCOS is thought to be excess insulin in the blood, which occurs as a result of insulin resistance.

Some of the signs and symptoms, such as fatigue, are a product of insulin resistance, whereas other symptoms are linked to the excess production of androgens from the ovaries and adrenal glands. Because androgen levels are out of whack, women with PCOS may develop conditions such as hirsutism and/or alopecia. Acne and obesity are other typical symptoms because of the increase in androgen. In one study of women seen in consultation primarily for acne, 45 percent of the cases were associated with polycystic ovaries.

It is apparent from this rainbow of symptoms that PCOS is not just a disease of the ovaries, it affects the whole body. For instance, because it causes one's periods to become irregular, women may be at greater risk for developing *endometrial hyperplasia*, where the uterine lining thickens to the point of becoming precancerous. (If you have endometrial hyperplasia, you may be given progesterone supplements to induce a period, or a procedure called a D&C to remove the endometrial lining.) Because of the high levels of androgens, women may also be at an increased risk for cardiovascular disease and therefore a heart attack.

ASSOCIATED HEALTH RISKS

PCOS is a risk factor for many serious medical conditions, so it is important to minimize symptoms as early as possible. PCOS can increase the risk of developing the following:

- Type 2 diabetes
- Coronary artery disease
- Stroke
- Early miscarriage (in the first trimester) or multiple miscarriages
- Multiple pregnancies (being pregnant with twins or more)
- High blood pressure
- Preeclampsia (a disorder that occurs in pregnancy, characterized by high blood pressure and protein in urine)
- Depression
- Fatty liver disease not associated with alcoholism
- Serious sleep disorders
- Uterine cancer
- Metabolic syndrome, also known as syndrome X
- Alzheimer's disease

Unwanted Hair and Hirsutism

Although this is a long and serious list, it represents worst-case scenarios; conditions such as uterine cancer rarely develop, even in untreated cases of PCOS. Nevertheless, insulin resistance is on the rise in the United States, as well as obesity, and there are correlations with PCOS. A full 50 percent of the population is insulin resistant, a condition in which the body resists normal functions of the hormone insulin. Insulin resistance and PCOS are major health hazards for women of all ages. Even lean women with PCOS can be insulin resistant, although weight gain can worsen their insulin resistance.

If you are shocked by this information, and perhaps are experiencing or have experienced some of these symptoms, you are not alone. Dr. Nadir Farid, a PCOS expert and coauthor of *The PCOS Diet Cookbook: Easy and Delicious Recipes & Tips for Women with PCOS on the Low GI Diet* (Farid and Gilletz, 2007), reports on his Web site, www.diagnosemefirst.com:

> PCOS is more than just a personal problem because it affects so many women. Due to its impact on different body functions, PCOS is a serious public health issue that deserves community support.

It certainly would be wise for policy makers and citizens to start paying attention to what is going on in women's bodies and make some public health and prevention strategies. The good news is that PCOS is treatable. A program that includes medications to sensitize the body to insulin, as well as lifestyle changes that address the signs and symptoms of PCOS, can be remarkably effective. Before discussing the treatment, let's look at how the ovaries become polycystic, how PCOS is diagnosed, what may cause it, and who is prone to it, including a look at the endocrine functions that are malfunctioning in women with PCOS.

Changes in the Ovaries

When a woman develops PCOS, it is due to excess androgen levels that interfere with her cycle, counteracting the normal process. Her estrogen levels are fine, but the elevated androgen levels interfere with the follicle stimulating hormone (FSH) necessary to trigger progesterone. The result is that the egg developed each month as part of her cycle is never released and instead turns into a small, pea-size cyst on the ovary that produced it. Over time, cysts can develop on both ovaries.

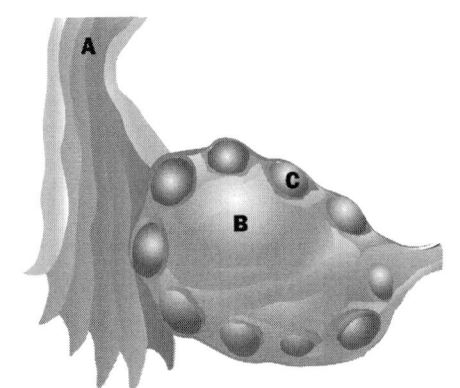

Figure 4. Illustration of an Polycystic Ovary

A. Fallopian tube
B. Polycystic ovary
C. Cyst (developing egg in healthy ovary)

Illustration by Kellie Frissell, www.kfdp.com

DIAGNOSING PCOS

A proper diagnosis will start you on your way to better health. Consulting a doctor trained to diagnosis PCOS may confirm your suspicions or set your mind at ease. A consultation may also diagnosis another disease associated with PCOS. In the meantime, because PCOS is associated with insulin, a hormone that regulates our blood sugar, you can start treating yourself by changing what you eat. Choose foods that contain complex carbohydrates (e.g., high-fiber breads, brown rice, semolina pasta, beans, and greens), which break down sugar slowly into your bloodstream, keeping your blood sugar more stable than other types of food. The Glycemic Index (GI) ranks carbohydrate foods according to the rate they raise blood glucose (sugar) levels during their absorption. Therefore, foods containing complex carbohydrates are called low glycemic index or low GI foods. A high GI diet contains a high level of simple carbohydrates (e.g., overly processed foods made with refined white flour, sugar, and corn syrup).

A low GI diet also reduces the onset of heart problems, which is a terrific secondary benefit. Sugar substitutes do not count; they actually make the problem worse. Do not make the common mistake of thinking that swapping fake sugar for real sugar will do the trick, no matter what the claims are in advertisements with beautiful women.

Unwanted Hair and Hirsutism

A PCOS diagnosis is made first by evaluating your history of acne, infertility, and menstruation; measuring your blood pressure, body mass index, and weight circumference; and observing hirsutism, acanthosis nigricans, hyperpigmentation, and alopecia. Not all patients satisfy the diagnostic criteria for this disease, therefore, it is important your doctor understands and suspects PCOS, before he or she orders blood tests and an ultrasound.

What the diagnostic blood tests look for are high levels of serum testosterone (a hormone), low levels of the sex hormone binding globulin (which is the protein that ferries testosterone and estrogens around the body), and high levels of lutenizing hormone (LH) compared to FSH. All very technical, but the good news is that it is possible to test these various hormone levels. An ultrasound of your ovaries that may identify a bulky ovary with ten or more peripheral cysts is also an indicator of PCOS.

If you are concerned that you may have PCOS and you are not ready to visit a doctor, you can take a quiz and answer a few questions yourself. To find out more and for a scoring system that will allow you to track these signs and symptoms, visit www.diagnosemefirst.com or the Polycystic Ovarian Syndrome Association (PCOA) at www.PCOSupport.org. When you are ready to set up a doctor's appointment, the PCOA and the American Association of Clinical Endocrinologists (AACE) at www.aace.com have a list of doctors specializing in PCOS.

CAUSES OF PCOS

Similar to many common disorders such as type 2 diabetes and heart disease, PCOS is known as a complex common trait, implying that lifestyle as well as genetic factors contribute to its development. These can include a diet that rates high on the glycemic index, little or no exercise, and stress.

Fat deposits—areas where fat cells accumulate—in the body differ according to location. Those in the midsection and inside the stomach are particularly sensitive to insulin, which induces an enzyme that converts steroid precursors into the hormone cortisol. Cortisol is often referred to as the "stress hormone" because stress also activates it; hence the findings that some people taking steroids are also insulin-dependent. Interestingly, research has shown that stress can induce changes in the body that lead to insulin resistance.

THE ROLE GENES PLAY IN PCOS
Some ethnic groups, such as indigenous peoples (e.g., American Indian, Aboriginal Australians, Pacific Islanders, or First Nations People in Canada), experience higher rates of both insulin resistance and PCOS than others do. Even in the general population, PCOS tends to run in families. Some research has shown that the PCOS trait seen in female family members may also show up in male members. Men experience this trait differently, however, usually displaying high serum dehydroepiandrosterone levels, weak adrenal androgen, high rates of frontal baldness, and central obesity. Sometimes, a woman with PCOS will also have a family history of diabetes, high blood pressure, or high cholesterol.

Recent research shows that genes implicated in PCOS are also involved in insulin action and in the production of sex hormones. It is actually the interrelationship among insulin resistance, ovarian hormones, and increased pituitary stimulation of the ovaries that account for all the symptoms and hormonal features of PCOS.

In addition, physiological changes associated with aging; for instance, the lower production of sex hormones, is also a factor in developing PCOS. Here again, stress and the resulting hormones play a role, accelerating aging processes.

THE ROLE INSULIN PLAYS IN PCOS
If your body develops a resistance to insulin, it compensates by producing excess hormones from the ovaries and adrenal glands, secreting more than average amounts of insulin. Insulin is a hormone essential for life; however, in excess amounts it causes a number of undesirable manifestations and symptoms, including PCOS. Excess insulin has a tendency to lay fats cells around the waist and inside the stomach, as well as to cause fat to infiltrate the muscles, liver, and even heart.

Excess insulin gradually compromises the ability of the pancreas to secrete insulin, to the extent that the pancreas simply cannot cope and you become insulin resistant, eventually developing diabetes.

A simple blood test that measures both insulin and *fasting glucose levels* helps diagnose insulin resistance. Before receiving the blood test you are instructed not to eat or drink anything but water for a certain amount of hours so the test can measure the sugar levels while you are fasting. Unfortunately, some research suggests that this blood test cannot diagnose at least 50 percent of the patients with PCOS. The results show that these patients have a normal fasting glucose/insulin relationship, although upon more technical investigation, are found to be insulin resistant.

Insulin does its job by latching onto a specific insulin receptor in your body. When it does, most of the receptor's concentration decreases, thus weakening the signal insulin transmits to the body's cells. Ovarian insulin receptors do not weaken, and thus your ovary is the target of persistent insulin action. Insulin both directly and indirectly stimulates the growth of the ovarian tissue between the eggs, which comprises the bulk of the ovary. Insulin also turns on the enzymes in the ovaries that make sex hormones. The sex hormone estrogen is made in the ovary through the conversion of testosterone. In PCOS, this conversion process is frequently malfunctioning, resulting in excess testosterone. It is this excess testosterone that causes hirsutism, abdominal weight gain, and possibly the development of male muscular features.

Excess insulin and testosterone also make the area at the base of the brain, known as the hypothalamus, more sensitive. As a result, the signal the hypothalamus sends to the pituitary gland becomes more frequent and intense. The pulses of luteinizing hormone that the pituitary secretes periodically become larger and more frequent. In a vicious cycle, the luteinizing hormone causes further ovarian stimulation and the oversecretion of sex hormones.

To make matters worse, insulin is responsible for converting weak sex hormones residing in the body's fat stores to more potent forms, again causing further symptoms such as hirsutism, acne, and frontal balding. Thus, the complex and chaotic interplay among the various glands of the endocrine system accounts for all of the symptoms of PCOS, which are further magnified by a high GI diet, no exercise, and stress.

MANAGING PCOS

PCOS needs to be identified and treated early so it does not progress because it predisposes a woman to serious health problems, including central obesity, fatty liver, and diabetes. But to manage PCOS successfully, you have to be prepared to make certain lifestyle changes. You will also have to stick with these changes to maintain good health and to control your PCOS. However, once you start making the changes, you may like how you feel and the way you look, too. Start by setting small goals, seek support, and keep at it.

Although pharmaceutical drugs used to treat PCOS are regularly used to sensitize the body to different hormones circulating in the endocrine system, drugs alone have limited benefit and may only reduce a few symptoms, unless they are accompanied by exercise, stress reduction techniques, and eating low GI foods.

See the discussion of drug therapies at the end of this chapter.

Exercise and Stress Reduction

Exercise and stress can impact your hormone production and affect your body in a positive manner. For example, you may have heard of a runner's high. Exercising reduces your stress levels, and feeling less stressed often helps you get off the couch and go for a walk.

Yoga is a wonderful method to gently exercise and stretch your body as well as rejuvenate your mind, body, and spirit. If you have never been much of an athlete, the gentle stretching is also a great way to learn how your body moves and breathes. Yoga can be done at an individual pace so you don't have to worry about keeping up with the class. Research classes and yoga centers to find one most in tune with your specific needs.

Walking is another great way to start exercising. There's no need to begin by running, even if you were a star athlete in high school. Walk alone or with a friend or family member. Adopting a dog can get you walking a few times a day, too. Dogs are also shown to reduce human stress, and they can be so affectionate!

Joining a support group, like the one at www.soulcysters.net (a support group for women with PCOS), may help relieve stress and anxiety. You can also find information about doctors and health insurance there.

Eating the Low Glycemic Index Way

One of the important influences of a low GI diet is that it positively effects the body's capacity to secrete insulin. A high GI diet causes large peaks of insulin secretion by the pancreas, whereas low GI eating results in a steady secretion of insulin. On a high GI diet you might experience sugar crashes. After a meal, you may become tired or sleepy, and then a few hours later become very hungry, resulting in the need to eat more to keep your blood sugar stable.

Unwanted Hair and Hirsutism

The glycemic index is a tool that ranks foods with a value of 0 to 100 according to their effect on blood sugar levels. Blood sugar changes produced by a given food are measured against the rise in blood sugar produced by a load of sugar (the chemical name is sucrose), which is 100 percent. To qualify as low GI, foods should have an index of 60 percent or less; those above 60 percent are considered high GI.

It is no surprise that traditional foods around the world are often associated with low GI foods, and that people who eat them or who ate them years ago generally were within a normal weight range, and not facing obesity like the U.S. population. Name your culture and find a low GI food, such as seminola wheat in Italy, black beans in the Caribbean, fava beans in the Middle East, basmati rice in India, couscous in northern Africa, plain yogurt in Greece, sticky rice in Japan, black bread in Germany, hard cheeses in Spain, or potatoes in Peru. You can find a list on the official Web site of the Glycemic Index and GI Database at www.glycemicindex.com.

It is also no surprise that many traditional foods are acidic or combine an acid flavor with other tastes: Think of sweet-and-sour sauce, tomato sauce, vinegar-based and wine sauces, widespread use of lemon in Latin America and the Middle East, fruits cooked with meat in Malaysia and Hungry, pickled herring in northern Europe, sauerkraut in Germany. Acid causes your stomach to empty slowly and therefore to digest and turn into sugar more slowly.

Foods processed and packaged and sold for quick eats significantly alter natural food and change its GI rating. For example, traditionally cooked oatmeal is highly touted for its health benefits; however, these nutritional benefits do not transfer to instant oatmeal. In fact, when the foods are processed, the grains or other ingredients convert into starches, which enter the bloodstream more rapidly. So even though natural oats cook fast, some cereal manufacturers have decided they need to cook quicker and have a variety of flavors, so they have processed the oats, added artificial flavors, and then packaged them. Many other companies also offer quick-cooking foods such as potatoes, rice, couscous, and vegetables.

The best rule of thumb is to keep away from processed foods (or most foods in a can, ready-to-eat-bag, or a box) and fast-food chains. Frozen vegetables cook just as easily covered in a microwave with your own olive oil and a clove of garlic as do the vegetables packaged in microwavable plastic bags and loaded with sodium, additives, and saturated oils. Avoid any foods with a long list of ingredients on the label, even if the product claims to be "natural." For example, maltodextrin, which has a high GI, is added to many foods, including popular brands of wheat bread. Currently, there is a movement in this country to make food labels more honest, which is being heavily lobbied against by the food manufacturers, who continue to flood the markets with more packaged foods.

Even some seemingly healthy foods cultivated in the United States have decreased in nutritional value, for example, corn, which once powered the ancient Mayan civilization with low-calorie protein, now rarely contains protein when grown in the United States. To make matters worse, corn syrup is processed to make high-fructose corn syrup, which replaces sugar in many processed foods and beverages (e.g., salad dressing, soda, crackers, and tomato sauce). Critics of high-fructose corn syrup point to its use and the increasing obesity rates in the United States. To find out more about corn grown in the United States and its damaging nutritional composition, watch the 2006 documentary *Corn Is King*, by filmmakers Aaron Woolf, Curt Ellis, and Ian Cheney.

The First Step to Eating Well

Learning how to shop is often the first obstacle to eating well. Many health food stores and co-ops offer free seminars on food and shopping tips. Also, farmers' markets are a great place to buy fresh foods that taste so good you don't need extra flavoring. And if you are lucky enough to live near a farm stand, stock up! You can buy in bulk and freeze vegetables, raw or cooked, in freezer bags or plastic containers. A movement gaining popularity is community-supported agriculture (CAS). A CAS program buys fresh vegetables and fruit in bulk from local farms and distributes them to its members on a regular basis. The choice of products is more limited than in a supermarket, but the food is fresh, not picked before it ripens, or frozen, and then shipped. The fresh food is tasty and inexpensive. The Web site www.localharvest.org has a list of places to find CSA programs near you. Organic meat is still expensive, so if you can't raise your own chickens, you can still get all the protein you need from meat by consuming smaller amounts. Certain types of fish and shellfish are still very inexpensive.

Here is one interesting experiment to do in a Chinese restaurant: Often the cooks and servers eat in the main dining room; if you go for a late dinner or lunch, watch what they serve themselves. You see big plates piled high with vegetables, lots of rice, and small amounts of meat. Then see what they serve non-Chinese customers: large plates of meat and small amounts of vegetables, generally swimming in cornstarch-laden sauces, and a small bowl of rice. Who can blame them for catering to U.S. tastes? Seek out restaurants with many Chinese patrons and/or try dim sum (traditional Chinese food served in small portions) on the weekends. These changes are happening across the board in previously traditional cuisine. You do not need to go to Little Italy to find pizzas covered in artery-hardening meats and extra cheeses, you can find them at most major chains and local pizzerias.

For great ideas on how to shop, snack, and cook the low GI way, get a copy of *The PCOS Diet Cookbook* (Farid and Gilletz 2007) published by Your Health Press and available at Amazon.com. Sharing a good meal and a walk afterward with a friend is a great way not only to practice your cooking, but to deepen a friendship and start new ones. Try inviting friends and neighbors to a potluck dinner.

The obesity epidemic in the United States over the last three decades has coincided with an overall increased intake of carbohydrate-containing, processed foods, with lower intakes of fiber. Fiber is a physical barrier that slows the absorption of carbohydrates into your bloodstream. Second- and even first-generation Latinos in the United States are a great case study. Instead of eating tortillas made from locally grown corn in their country of origin, many U.S. Latinos eat white-flour tortillas and snack on soda and chips instead of fibrous fruits and vegetables. Their rates of diabetes and heart disease are sky rocketing. This is not to say that Mexico isn't experiencing a similar obesity problem in recent years, but the contrast in one generation in the United States is astounding.

What has made matters worse in the United States is our tendency to eat one or two large meals a day. This results in tsunami-size insulin peaks, which predispose us to weight gain, as well as a host of symptoms and side effects that result from excess insulin in the blood. Fat stores around the midriff (often called "belly fat") are especially sensitive to the effects of insulin, therefore, too much insulin makes it exceedingly difficult for the body to use abdominal fat as a source of fuel because one of its functions is to inhibit the release of fat from fat stores. When fat accumulates gradually around the midsection of girls or women, it is typically a sign of PCOS, but more generally a sign of insulin resistance in both women and men.

To address these symptoms and side effects, it is necessary to regularly eat a diet of healthy low GI foods to maintain low levels of insulin in the blood. If you have PCOS, low GI eating can help reduce your symptoms and halt the progression of your disease. It can also decrease insulin levels, making it easier for your body to burn fat.

Other advantages to a low GI diet, include:

- Lowering your blood fats (or triglycerides)
- Enabling you to feel fully satisfied after eating
- Reducing your risk of developing diabetes and other diseases
- Improving your physique (as your body redistributes its fat stores, you will lose belly fat and weight)
- Allowing for better-quality sleep
- Improving your overall sense of well-being

Drug Therapies

In some women with PCOS, excess androgens cause many symptoms and interfere with insulin regulation. Your doctor may want to put you on a corticosteroid to suppress your adrenal gland and therefore lower your body's production of androgens. This also helps to induce ovulation.

Oral hypoglycemic agents used to treat type 2 diabetes are being used to treat PCOS by lowering insulin, which may help to restore your menstrual cycle and lower androgen levels. Research has found this treatment to be effective even in women who are not insulin resistant or obese.

However, before you're placed on an insulin-lowering drug, ask your doctor about the ways in which diet and exercise can help your body use insulin more efficiently. Also ask how insulin-lowering drugs may affect your ability to become pregnant and about any side effects.

Women who are diabetic, or who have a problem with their adrenal glands, thyroid gland, or pituitary gland, can develop symptoms of PCOS without technically having the condition. Ask your doctor to rule out the conditions involving these glands before you begin any treatment for PCOS. In some cases, PCOS may coincide with these conditions.

Unwanted Hair and Hirsutism

If PCOS is caught early in your menstrual history, you may be prescribed a combination oral contraceptive (referred to as a birth control pill). The effects of oral contraception therapy regulate hormone production (which is how it prevents pregnancy). This regulation induces your body's natural bleeding by adjusting your endocrine system so that it produces normal levels of estrogen and progesterone.

Or you may be put on progestin, a synthetic progesterone supplement that also regulates your system. If you were treated with progestin at a young age for irregular cycles, you won't experience problems with your cycle unless you stop taking it. However, you may not know why you suffered from irregular periods in the first place. When women go off contraceptives to conceive, they are plagued by the same symptoms that warranted oral contraceptives initially, but now they have the added difficulty of conceiving.

If you are struggling with infertility, diet alone is not considered a realistic short-term treatment because the positive effects can be gradual. However, if you are being treated with fertility drugs, you may aid your fertility with natural methods as described earlier. Consult with a nutritionist to design a program to help you become pregnant.

CHAPTER 6

HAIR: WHAT STIMULATES IT AND WHAT KILLS IT

Now that you know about the hormones that make hair grow, if you understand how it grows, you will be better equipped to decide how to remove it.

Figure 5. Hair Follicle

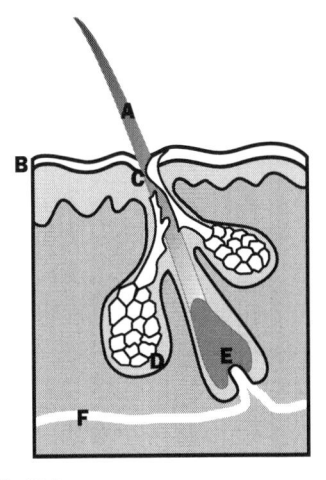

A. Hair shaft
B. Skin layer
C. Pore
D. Sebaceous gland
E. Hair root
F. Blood vessel

© 2009 Your Health Press

    The hair root is what we cannot see; it is below the skin's surface inside the hair follicle—which we never see. When you pluck the hair, the darker, bulbous point you see is called a root. Because the root comes from a hair follicle that stays within the skin, when you pluck or yank out a hair, you are not getting rid of that follicle's ability to grow the next hair. The cells in the bottom third of the follicle, in particular the dermal papilla, just generate new ones as the hair cycles through. What is even worse is that the hair may grow in coarser and darker depending on how much the removal method aggravates the skin and hair follicle.

Unwanted Hair and Hirsutism

Since hair is designed to protect the skin from harsh elements, when you irritate the skin with hot wax or other hair removal chemicals, your body's response will be to nourish the follicles with blood, thereby strengthening your hair. Blood flow helps to determine hair growth, too, which is why some people may have more hair on one side than on the other.

The skin wants to keep its protector—the hair—and therefore uses its other appendages to nurture and baby the hair follicle to keep it healthy. Our sebaceous glands lubricate and protect the hair. (This is one of the reasons why oily skin often accompanies excessive, unwanted hair.)

Hair is sensitive to environmental temperatures and grows more rapidly when you feel hot because of increased blood flow to the epidermis, a typical aggravation for women who want to go to the beach without dark hair on their legs.

You probably know that skin is constantly renewing itself; as dead skin cells slough off, new ones are created. The same thing occurs with hair, as you've noticed when washing your hair. You have a normal amount of hair that you lose each week. In fact, if you notice an increased hair loss, it indicates something is not quite right in your body, and taken into account with other symptoms, probably leads to a doctor's diagnosis of a medical problem. Pregnancy also causes you to lose hair on your head a few months after pregnancy, but this is after delivery when your androgen levels are returning to normal. This is temporary and normal.

Hair falls out, but it also grows again for its genetically programmed amount of time. Growth cycles vary for hair on different parts of our body. After menopause we lose hair that is dependent on androgens to trigger its growth, basically our terminal hair. You'll notice the numbers of hair thinning in general, as hair that falls out is not replaced in that follicle.

If you can't wait for that day to come, or if you are now growing hair in new areas, the next chapters describe methods to remove it. There are two types of hair removal. *Depilation* removes the hair shaft from the skin's surface and *epilation* removes hair from the follicle. Depilation effects, such as from shaving and creams, usually only last for a maximum of a few days. Epilation methods—such as plucking, waxing, or other methods that extract hairs to above the bulb—last longer. Epilation can cause hyperpigmentation of the skin, particularly in women of color.

To date, the only way to permanently prevent a hair from growing is to kill the cells in the hair follicle. This is done through electrolysis, a hair-by-hair technique described further in chapter 9.

Removing hair by any means, but more so by epilation, can cause inflamed hair follicles. Any further irritation or friction can cause the area to become infected and afflicted with a condition called folliculitis. It appears as tiny, pimple like bumps that become red and puffy and can eventually scar your skin.

Folliculitis forms a cyst of pus as your white blood cells are irritated. Many women, often those with dark skin or with coarse, curly hair, often experience ingrown hairs and folliculitis because of repeated tweezing, shaving, plucking, picking, or waxing. This can lead to skin discoloration (darker) and the development of keloids (scar tissue on the surface of the skin). Be careful not to shave or pick at the infection. Folliculitis can be especially painful in the bikini area, which your underwear may hit up against. It can lead to keloids, particularly among women of color, which are permanent and shiny.

Ingrown hairs are troublesome as a result of any type of hair removal. This happens when hair grows back into the skin causing large, painful bumps. It occurs more frequently to people with curly hair. It is more common in the pubic hair region and especially painful where there is friction from skin rubbing together and against underwear and pants. If you pick at an ingrown hair, you could scar your skin.

If your follicles are inflamed, which you will often see after shaving, leave them alone. Don't put chemicals on your skin and beware of commercial lotions and oils with fragrances and chemicals. Cold compresses and pure aloe helps treat a case of razor burn. Warm compresses and removing external irritants can help with pain from folliculitis while you heal. Electrolysis can remove the infection.

REAL WOMEN GROW HAIR

If you have hirsutism or hypertrichosis, or are ethnically hairier than your peers from northern European decent, it does not mean you are more male-like or less feminine than your less hairy peers. Nor does it mean you are lesbian.

Why? First, as discussed in chapter 2, whether or a terminal hair grows is affected by skin cells. We all have skin, males and female alike, and I'm sure you've noticed how similar skin is for everyone.

Second, it is a misnomer to associate testosterone and other androgens

Unwanted Hair and Hirsutism

only with men. Women have them, and must have them. The same can be said of estrogens. The dichotomy of women versus men is not accurate. We are not polar opposites. Our body is more similar than different, and vastly similar at that. Therefore, if your body produces more terminal hair than other women do, it does not make you manly. It just makes you hairier.

Third, there's plenty of evidence that levels of androgen, in particular testosterone, are not predictive of hair growth, especially in its lower levels. Yes, there is a correlation for hyperandrogenemia and tumors, but a tumor does not make a woman a man or a man a woman. It means you have a tumor. You have read in earlier chapters how hyperandrogenemia is a symptom of many medical conditions and how hirsutism is correlated with those levels. However, hormones fluctuate widely in your body during puberty, adolescence, pregnancy, and menopause. These changes are normal and an increase in androgen levels, at any level, does not change you into a man.

In addition, there are plenty of incidences where a woman will have hirsutism and not have an unusually high amount of androgens or an increase in them.

It is certainly part of the mainstream culture for women who have dark body hair, muscles, a broad body, or who are tall to be stereotyped as masculine. It is not so long ago that women with a broad body were desirable for their strength, fortitude, and childbearing potential.

This is not a whole lot of comfort if you struggle with your self-identity as a woman, but it does put in perspective some notions of what a woman should look like. You also might gain some perspective by seeking out role models of women with whom you find a physical connection. Unfortunately, most women who appear in the news, even those who are not in the entertainment business, are also "adjusted" for television or photos. If you can't travel to the region of your ancestry, the Internet has all kinds of media from all over the world and might be a source of images of women similar to you (just be aware of what publications you look at, however; many countries such as Argentina and Korea have higher rates of plastic surgery than does the United States, so they probably have high rates of photographing women as stereotypical images). If you are lucky enough to have grandmothers or great-aunts whom you see regularly, who immigrated to the United States or Canada, try not to judge them against the mainstream cultural values, but instead look to see how they view themselves as women.

CHAPTER 7

HAIR REMOVAL METHODS

When I was 10 or 11, I was so self-conscious about my hairy legs that I spent one whole summer avoiding the pool deck, in the water as much as possible. If I had to sit out, I wrapped a towel around my legs as I sat in a deck chair. My mother finally relented and allowed me to shave my legs. That first shave was thrilling. —C.F.

Hair removal has become a rite of passage for women in the United States. When you finally get your parents' permission to shave, you feel all grown up. It is ironic that once your body enters adulthood, society says to revert back to looking like a child. Talk about sending mixed messages. However, if you are navigating this culture, you likely find times when you want to remove your hair. Now that you know more about hair growth, you can make an educated decision about which methods work best for you.

Methods of removing unwanted hair depend on where it is growing and the quantity. Plus, not all women want the same level of removal. Our tolerances depend on many cultural and practical factors, such as where we live, the time of year, or pressure from our partners—equally influenced by our culture and what he or she thinks is attractive. Maybe you can share your newfound knowledge from this book with your partner. Or perhaps a potential partner's tolerance or intolerance of your natural and normal hair growth helps or hinders your ability to form a nurturing relationship. Suprisingly, many women find that contrary to what we have learned, many men care far less about our hair than we do! Other factors include cost as well as time and convenience in this chapter.

This chapter also warns of potential product scams. Although hair removal is a hugely popular and lucrative industry, generally it is not regulated by the Federal Drug Administration (FDA). In fact, the FDA does not regulate many products in general. This means that you can buy almost any product in stores and on the Internet that claim to remove hair or stop hair growth. Products approved by the FDA advertise this fact. If the packaging does not say that the product is approved by the FDA, then it is not. "FDA-approval pending" means the product is still being tested and is a safer bet than products

Unwanted Hair and Hirsutism

without FDA approval. It is important to do your own research and shop in local food co-ops or natural food stores that evaluate products before they sell them. Even then, ask questions as many remedies still promise big and deliver little, and some have proven to be harmful.

Before you remove any unwanted hair, consider the following factors:

1. *Can you get ahead of the game?* If you have a hormonal problem, it will be difficult to "get ahead of the game" because your hair follicles are constantly being stimulated by the androgens. You can remove the hair shaft (the part you see), but depending on the androgen activity in your skin cells, the hair might come back very quickly.

   Serious underlying conditions are atypical. If you think you may have a hormonal imbalance, many of the hair removal methods listed here can be considered once the underlying hormonal problem causing the excessive or unwanted hair growth has been ruled out. With your doctor's consultation, combine your treatment with one or more of the hair removal choices described in this chapter. Hirsutism may end when you take care of the underlying problem. See chapter 3 for more information on the causes of hirsutism.

2. *Normal fluctuations*, such as those caused by your monthly cycle, are common reasons for hair growth. Most often, fluctuating hormone levels are to blame for the appearance of a moustache, chin hairs, belly-button hair, or other hairs. During certain parts of your menstrual cycle, your hair darkens. During these darker-hair days, try different hairstyles, lipstick shades, and shirt colors to detract from unwanted hair on your face. Skip the midriff tops and low-rise jeans or wear a bathing suit with a skirt to conceal the darker hairs on your inner thighs. You just may be able to tolerate the dark hair for a few days rather than running to wax.

   If you feel self-conscious around your partner or someone you are dating, go ahead and bring it up, at least you will not continue worrying if he or she notices. Chances are he is not so oblivious as to not have noticed his mother's darkening upper lip periodically. And if your partner is a she, then she has the same issues as you do. Even if her hair darkens to a lesser degree, it may still bother her the same as

Unwanted Hair and Hirsutism

it does you. And don't be fooled into thinking that fair-haired women don't have the same issues. Even if you're a dark-haired woman and haven't noticed darker hair growth on your fair friends during particular days of the menstrual cycle, they surely have. It's all relative!

People often notice when you are suddenly hairless, so if you rush to remove the hair on your upper lip, people still may think something looks out of place on you. We are so accustomed to thinking that hair is bad, when in reality our friends and colleagues have an image of us, hair and all. Rarely do people dissect friends and significant others part by part (and if they do, you may want to reconsider that relationship).

3. *A temporary trial,* before you try electrolysis allows you to see how you like the hairless look. Electrolysis does not just get rid of the dark hair that you don't like contrasting against your skin it removes the whole hair from that follicle. You may decide after electrolysis that your face, leg, or stomach looks bald without hair, and you don't like that, either. There is no going back.

This chapter summarizes the hair removal methods currently on the market, so you can make an informed decision. It also describes the best methods for specific areas of the body, such as side effects, average costs, and general convenience. Separate chapters are devoted to electrolysis (chapter 9) and to laser treatment (chapter 10).

SHAVING

You have probably always heard that one of the worst ways to remove hair is by shaving. And it certainly seems true because when we shave the hair appears to grow back thicker and coarser. However, that stubbly feeling is simply the result of cutting the hair at its thickest point—the remainder of the hair strand then has a blunt feeling. Although shaving causes the hair to grow back faster as compared to yanking methods such as waxing, threading, sugaring, stringing, electronic devices, and tweezing, shaving *does not increase* the hair follicle's growth rate or strengthen it as these methods do, because it does nothing to affect the actual follicle.

Shaving also does not cause hair to thicken, which is another common misconception. In fact, hirsutism experts and studies have shown that shaving cannot influence hair density in any way (yes, studies have been done!).

If your goal is to remove the hair without stimulating and further strengthening the roots, then shaving, believe it not, is better than yanking methods (see chapter 1). Shaving also will not make hirsutism worse than it already is. This will come as relief to many women who shave their legs and underarms, as well as to women who have shaved other parts of their body. Shaving is also a good way to exfoliate the skin, which can improve its texture.

If your goal, however, is to remove the hair so it stays away for a long time and does not grow back stubbly, then shaving is not a good method. Shaving is not recommended for your eyebrows or arms, and it can be problematic for curly hair, which is prone to becoming ingrown. Shaving is also questionable for your pubic area.

Shaving can cause other problems, such as razor burn (raised and puffy red bumps), ingrown hair, and folliculitis, which are especially painful in the groin, bikini, and pubic areas. This is because pants and underwear rub against the tender skin.

If you get ingrown hairs after shaving, never run a razor over them. You can cut and possibly scar your skin or cause folliculitis. You can cause changes in your pigmentation as well. If ingrown hairs are common for you, try another hair removal method or reduce the number of times you shave each month, especially if you shave by habit, whether or not anyone sees your legs. If you shave because you don't like your hair, try keeping it intact for a while and see if you can change the way you feel about yourself. You may decide you don't "have" to shave so frequently after all.

A triple-blade razor gives a faster, cleaner shave than the less expensive single or double blades, or those marketed to women with sensitive skin. If you have coarse or thick hair, try men's razors. Also, use shaving cream for men as it may be more effective at holding your hair in the razor's way than women's creams. Follow the directions on the shaving cream bottle for the best shave, and never shave dry or without lubrication. The cheap, single-blade razors require that you run it over your skin more times, making the skin prone to cuts and folliculitis. In general, don't use a disposable blade more than a few times and never use it if it is getting rusty.

For the closest shave, do not shave after first waking, as the skin tends to be swollen. Also, shave against the direction of hair growth unless you are prone to razor burn or folliculitis. For sensitive areas such as the bikini line, shave in the direction of hair growth. Be sure to use a moisturizing lubricant afterward. For tiny cuts or irritation, use an antibacterial cream, aloe (use the aloe leaf itself or pure bottled aloe; avoid the many brands that contain other irritants), or a medicated lotion to soothe.

If the hair on your legs is long, shaving may cause a lot of irritation and take a lot of time because the longer hairs are easily caught in the blade. Cut the hair with scissors first or use a hair removal cream and then follow up the next day or as needed with a razor. Use small, sharp scissors made for haircutting. A good primer on shaving is in the book *Body Drama* (Redd 2008).

Electronic razors are becoming more high-tech all the time. Some automatically dispense lotion. Others are waterproof and can be used in the shower. Mostly marketed to men, you can find a few for women. You may, however, prefer those marketed to men if you find one more effective and easier to manipulate.

An endocrinologist may encourage shaving in combination with hormone therapy as it helps determine whether the hair growth is decreasing (by counting the number of days between shaves). An electrologist may encourage shaving first to show which hairs are in the anagen phase of growth (where destruction is most effective) so these hair strands can be permanently removed early in treatment.

Cost and Convenience

Shaving with disposable razors is cheap and convenient as long as you have water and soap. Triple-blade razors are more expensive than single blades, but men's shaving products in general are cheaper than those marketed to women. There are plenty of coupons available for extra savings, and generic brands are usually significantly cheaper than brand names. Pure aloe is more expensive than the blends you will find at the big stores, but you'll notice the difference in its soothing ability, plus you'll have it on hand for burns and cuts.

Shaving with an electronic razor requires purchasing a razor for anywhere from $20 to $300. If the razor is battery operated, it will require a periodic added expense and hassle unless you have one that is rechargeable. Electronic razors are almost as convenient as disposable ones if you have electricity available, but they are heavier. Men's electronic razors are also generally cheaper than those for women, which are hard to find.

Unwanted Hair and Hirsutism

Shaving can be time-consuming and if you do it in the shower, it necessitates running water. If you have a bathroom setup where you can sit and shave and then rinse, you'll save energy. If your partner is keen on shaved legs, make him do it in the bath with you and he'll see how long it takes. Perhaps his "I have to shave every day" will contrast with the amount of time it takes to shave two legs at often awkward positions without a mirror. But it can be an excuse to get in the tub together and save water.

TRIMMERS AND GROOMING KITS

Trimmers are small electronic devices that are marketed for trimming stray hairs, last-minute hair strands that escape other removal methods and sparse or, small body areas For example, after you have shaved your legs, you undoubtedly notice some stray ankle hairs. Some trimmers are marketed to "clean up" eyebrows. The reviews of these products are not good. The cheaper ones in particular seem to lose their battery charge easily. Many are waterproof. Check product reviews before purchasing and consider scissors or manual trimmers instead.

Grooming kits usually come with a trimmer, scissors, different size combs, tweezers, and other devices. Women's kits are more expensive than those for men. Men's kits also have nose clippers, which women's don't (seems like an oversight by the marketing folks!). Kits for women can be $100 whereas a comparable one for men is $40. If you have several grooming needs, the kits are cost-effective. They are also great when you are traveling or have meetings and you notice some pesky hairs that you didn't see in the morning.

LASER RAZOR

Although there has been a stir about this product that purportedly to zaps away your hair permanently or for long periods of time—mainly because of a *Wired* magazine article a few years ago—this product does not exist. Do not be fooled into buying the laser razor on the Internet, because all of the advertisements are scams. The technology does not exist.

Gillette states that it has FDA approval for an in-home laser removal device, but it is not a razor. According to Gillette, the technology is a light-based hair remover developed in partnership with Palomar Medical Technologies, Inc. The device is only a prototype and the company has no plans to develop it.

TWEEZING

A one-time investment in a good pair of sturdy tweezers that are easy to manipulate ranges from $10 to $30. The cheaper ones are made of flimsy material and often the ends don't match up well enough to grab the hair. Tweezing is generally considered a good method to use on your eyebrows, since you may want to change the shape from time to time and allow the hair to grow back.

Tweezing sparse facial hairs on the chin, out of moles, around your nipples, on your upper lip area, on your toes, under your belly button, or elsewhere on your body can give you immediate short-term gratification—followed by long-term aggravation when the hair grows back stronger and coarser, generally worsening your hair problem. Scar tissue can also form during tweezing, which may be as undesirable as the original hair, or may make the eyebrow shape a permanent feature.

Over tweezing or digging too deep with tweezers can cause your skin to look pitted. Be very careful when tweezing and don't break your skin to remove an ingrown hair, let it grow out naturally. Use a loofah sponge or exfoliator to remove dead skin cells that may be blocking a hair.

Some women tweeze for years and don't mind doing so as they continue to deal with the same few hairs they know well. However, if you have more than a few hairs, tweezing may not be for you because the hair keeps coming back. Tweezing is a terrible way to remove large areas of unwanted hair.

ELECTRIC TWEEZERS

None of the claims that electric tweezers painlessly remove hair or result in permanent hair removal are true. The electric tweezer industry is growing in the United States, and the devices now are used regularly in salons, which advertise the service as permanent. It isn't.

This is how it works: the tweezers grasp a hair strand and run a current through it. Because you have to hold the hair in the grasp of the tweezers to deliver the current, it is much slower than manual tweezing, contrary to claims for a "fast tweeze."

The best areas for using electric tweezers are underarms or areas with sparsely growing hair. The results are short term and can cause infections and ingrown hairs. You may damage a few hair follicles along the way to the point the hair can't grow back (and hopefully you won't get ingrown hair), although the pain and lack of permanence is hardly worth it. Because the hair is yanked out, the devices also strengthen the hair follicle, encouraging hair growth.

Electric tweezers are often marketed for ones' breasts and face but, again, the results are short term and may worsen the problem over the long term. Never use these products on your arms, as this will only make the hair growth problem worse.

Cost and Convenience

Electric tweezers range from $20 to $100. As with other methods of epilation, some women don't feel too much pain after using them a few times or can tolerate it. But if you generally feel pain with epilation methods, you might find spending money on this device a waste.

There is no substantiation that electric tweezers marketed as professional tweezers used by salons are any better than personal ones, and they are much more expensive. The wide range of prices does not reflect value. Remember, this is an unregulated industry, so there is no way to justify the claims objectively. While customer reviews on Web sites are not objective, they can give one an idea about a product.

One claim made by companies that sell electric tweezers is that they are an alternative to electrolysis. Just because they zap you with electricity does not make them similar to electrolysis. Electrolysis is permanent; electric tweezers do not remove hair permanently. Stay away from any product if the retailer advertises its permanency. If the company lies about this feature, it is probably lying about the product's other features as well.

These tweezers are convenient if you have electricity and don't have many hairs to tweeze. Many women prefer to tweeze in the bathroom, so remember that these are electric devices and be careful, as with any electrical device, near water.

EPILATORS

These devices round up your hair with an electronic spinning motion and yank it out. Epilators are notoriously painful, and most women find they can't tolerate these devices. They also can cause skin irritation and sensitivity, leading to folliculitis or ingrown hairs. And like any method of yanking, epilators strengthen the follicle. Hair removal is temporary and, like regular tweezing, stimulates the hair follicles to grow stronger hair. If hair doesn't grow back, it is because you have created scar tissue in the follicle.

These electronic devices entered the market in the 1980s and are relatively cheap and convenient, although expensive brands are also offered. There is no difference among the brands' effectiveness because they all yank your hair out, so here again, do not be fooled by companies, stating their brand is "professional" or like those used in salons.

These are not recommended to use near hair you do not want to remove because the epilator could easily grab vellus hair or other hair in the vicinity. Also, do not use these on your eyebrows, upper lip, pubic area, or any other area near sensitive skin.

Epilators range in price from $35 to $120. Some devices use batteries and are convenient for traveling, but be prepared for a $25 expense for a battery that requires replacement.

HAIR REMOVAL CREAM

Hair removal cream does less damage to the hair follicle than does epilation and does not worsen hirsutism as epilation methods do.

Hair removal cream works by chemically dissolving the hard keratin of the hair shaft so that the hair does not grow back stubbly as it does with shaving. The active ingredients in most creams are thioglycolates, which disrupt disulfide bonds in the hair. You'll notice that they smell a little bit like sulfur.

To use the cream, spread a small amount onto the hair you want to remove and wait three to ten minutes, depending on the instructions, then wash away the hair. If you wait too long, you can burn your skin (feels similar to dying your hair). After waiting the instructed time in the directions, you can calculate future time according to your hair and success at removal. It is easiest to do before you jump in the shower. While the pressure from the water loosens most of the cream and hair, briskly running your hands over the areas or using a washcloth or bath sponge will remove the rest. Be sure to remove all of the cream from your body.

Cream is great for long hair and is a lot quicker than shaving. If you are prone to razor burn or ingrown hairs, hair removal cream is a good choice. Using a hair catcher in the tub is a good idea if you are removing a lot of hair.

One downside of hair removal cream is that it may irritate the soft keratin of your skin. The chemicals can cause contact dermatitis in some people. Test for any negative reactions by applying cream to a small area on your leg first. Use a thick moisturizing cream afterward, such as Aquaphor, Eucerin (or their generic equivalents), pure shea butter, or pure aloe if you are prone to dry skin or eczema.

Hair removal cream is not recommended for your pubic area because the cream can easily spread to your vaginal area during the waiting period (although creams now work within minutes) or showering. It is best used on areas that are completely covered with terminal hair, such as the bottom parts of your legs, inside thighs and underarms, or anywhere you have a patch of hair you want to remove, otherwise you risk taking off vellus hair as well. If you only have a few hairs to take off, it may be overtreating and you should consider the effect of putting chemicals on your skin where there is no bothersome hair. If you use a hair removal cream on your face, use it very carefully and far from your eyes, nostrils, and mouth; and don't walk around with the product on your face, to prevent the harsh chemicals from trickling into one of those areas.

Some hair removal creams are more effective than others, and some have more chemicals than others do. Manufacturers add fragrance to mask unpleasant odors. The more heavily fragranced, the more chemicals contained in the product that can potentially irritate your skin, as most beauty companies don't use real oils when they add fragrance.

If you have thick, coarse hair or sensitive skin, look for creams marketed to men for their facial hair. Often this is for African-American men and comes in a can that looks like shaving cream. As with many products and services, hair removal cream is cheaper for men than for women.

Cost and Convenience

The most popular brands are about $5 to $9 for a bottle the size of a can of men's large shaving cream, making it very inexpensive, especially if you use it in small areas. Depending on where and which brands you are buying, some of these creams also can be expensive. Small containers seem to be pricier than large ones, and are therefore more expensive per application, and cost as much as $50 for an ounce or two. Check the ingredients and you will see that the active chemicals are the same in the fancy small jars as they are in the bigger, cheaper bottles. Like many women's beauty products—fragrances, makeup, soap, or lotion—they are overpriced. Consult consumer sources to find the best cream for the best price.

Unwanted Hair and Hirsutism

As long as you have water, you can use a cream. An old towel might help during application. Keep the cream on the palms of your hands and fingertips or wash immediately after applying, so you won't risk removing the hair from the back of your hands. If you accidentally apply cream somewhere else on your skin, wash it off immediately, as the longer it stays on the more time the chemicals have to work.

GROWTH-INHIBITING CREAM

Some growth-inhibiting creams on the market purport to minimize or reduce hair growth over the course of treatment. At this writing, all the over-the-counter products (except Vaniqa, a prescribed cream) in stores or on the Internet are scamming you. These herbal products and growth-inhibiting creams are marketed from well-known cosmetic and specialty brands. They are fraudulent. In this case, there is no connection between well-known brands and quality, but somehow it has taken root in U.S. consciousness that popular companies must be looking after you. This is not true. None of these products work, no matter what claims the company makes or how well they advertise. This goes for herbal remedies, too. None of these creams are approved by the FDA, and they may cause contact dermatitis or otherwise irritate your skin. Do not waste your money or risk damaging your skin. If you feel compelled to try one, always do a spot test.

Vaniqa

Vaniqa is the only cream proven to reduce hair growth. It does not remove hair. For more information, see page 68. It is available by prescription only, unless you buy it in another country, in which case, be aware of the chemicals it contains, the approved age groups, and the side effects).

The FDA approved Vaniqa in 2000 for women over age twelve, and only for facial hair. It is a topical cream that inhibits hair growth through supplying an enzyme to your skin that interferes with the hair follicle and thus the hair's growth.

While testing Vaniqa for various other disorders, alopecia was found to be a side effect. Scientists find many unintentional uses for drugs this way. Vaniqa is actually an antiprotozoan drug that was originally developed for sleeping sickness. The chemical compound is eflornithine hydrochloride.

Unwanted Hair and Hirsutism

Cost and Convenience

Vaniqa costs about $115 per package. Each package has two tubes (you can buy just one) of 30 grams each, so they are rather small. When the drug is available generically in a few years, the cost will undoubtedly come down. If another cream is developed to compete with Vaniqa, perhaps the cost will be a bit lower as well. With a success rate of only 60 percent, there is a lot of room for a similar drug to be developed. The cream is very convenient as the tube is small to carry and it is a leave-on cream, therefore you don't need water or towels or anything else.

BLEACHING CREAM

Bleaching kits do not remove hair, they bleach the fine, dark, hairs on the upper lip or other areas to conceal hirsutism and unwanted hair. Some women find this works well. Bleaches contain hydrogen peroxide and sulfates, and have an unpleasant smell. Side effects include irritation, tiny red itchy bumps, and possible pigmentation changes, especially with olive or darker complexions.

Once the cuticle rises to allow the chemicals to bleach the hair, it never really lies all the way back down again after the bleach has done its job. The resulting hair may take on a stand-away-from-the-skin appearance. (As with the hair on your head, any dye or chemical application tends to cause a change in texture.)

Bleaching may change hair color to shades ranging from copper to blond. On olive-skinned women, the light hair may contrast with your skin and become more noticeable after bleaching than your original darker hairs!

Do not bleach your eyebrows or the hair near your vagina. The chemicals can be dangerous.

Bleaching is temporary, of course, and relates to the speed in which your hair grows. So if you are of Mediterranean descent, you will notice dark hair growing back faster in the area than it does for fairer women.

Cost and Convenience

Bleaching can be time consuming, but otherwise all you need is water, gloves, and a towel. Bleach (often sold in "kits" with applicators and aftercare lotion) run from $4 to $10 for an ounce or two. Only a tiny bit is needed for upper lip hair; however, it is more expensive for large areas of hair. Check the kit components; you already may have lotion, aloe, or oil in your bath or kitchen that you can apply afterward, and can buy just the bleach.

FRICTION

Have you ever noticed that you have less hair on your legs at the places where your jeans are the tightest? This is because friction removes the hair a little at a time. Some people use loofah sponges regularly to slowly wear away the hair. These sponges are marketed as skin exfoliators, not hair removal products, because it requires a lot of scrubbing to actually remove hair. Loofah sponges are natural gourds (squash family) that are dried and packaged. The natural, unbleached sponges are more effective because they are harder than the bleached ones. They are a natural a tan color. (If you see blue or green ones, they are treated with chemicals.) The loofah's cylindrical shape fits nicely under one's underarm and can loosen the hair there.

Several companies sell friction devices, such as a loofah mitt that you place over your hand and rub against your skin. The results are mixed. Some women report experiencing utter pain, whereas others say it works slowly but surely. It likely depends on your hair texture and the sensitivity of your skin, and is not recommended for sensitive areas. Common areas to use friction are on the tougher parts of your body, such as your legs. Friction is not yanking and does not simulate tweezing, therefore it doesn't hurt the hair follicle and thereby increase hair's toughness or growth.

Cost and Convenience

Most people use loofah sponges in the shower for normal bathing as a skin exfoliator or a washcloth, so they are very convenient. Using these devices as a regular method to remove hair, however, is extremely time consuming, if they work at all. Combining a friction device with other methods has some merit, although it could make the skin more sensitive if used just prior to applying cream, shaving, or other treatments.

Sold for pennies a piece in other countries, a loofah sponge can cost several dollars in the United States. Mitts cost a few dollars each. Keep these dry so they last longer and do not collect mildew.

BODY SUGARING

Sugaring involves applying a sticky substance to your skin and pressing it with cloth or paper strips. When you rip it off, the hair sticks to the substance and is pulled out. The best areas to sugar are the face, legs, and underarms. Sugaring can be messy and, as a result, is not convenient. A sugaring compound is available in some drugstores. One container lasts a long time and can be purchased for $10 to $50. Most sugaring kits are sold on television or through special offers. Be cautious about making a homemade concoction with honey and other ingredients because the "recipe" is not commonly available and is volatile according to temperature, types of honey used, and so on. Some states regulate professional sugaring at a salon. Beware when going to a salon that is not credentialed (see page 149 for information about regulations).

THREADING

Threading is an ancient technique often used in such places as India, China, and the Middle East. It is now becoming popular in the United States and Canada, especially in neighborhoods with many women from these other regions of the world. It is called by different names, for instance *khite* in Arabic and *fatlah* in Egyptian.

Threading involves the use of a regular cotton thread to remove hair from the surface of the skin. It requires a trained threading professional. The thread is tied around the practitioner's neck or between her teeth and looped around her fingers, and then quickly twisted across the surface of the skin. The practitioner pushes the string down while it spins, and when she pulls up, the string grabs the hair, pulling it out of the follicle as it moves. The up and down movement is repeated over the hair, even very short stubble.

Many women report that it is less painful than waxing or tweezing, but it can have the same side effects, including folliculitis and ingrown hairs. If you have sensitive skin, try it conservatively at first to see how your skin reacts, as it can be irritating. Threading does hurt the hair follicle.

Cost and Convenience

Threading is best for small areas, but it can be done on large areas, too. Costs are similar to waxing ($8 to $20 for eyebrows or upper lip). Larger body areas may cost up to $200. The advantage of threading is that it can massage the skin and the muscles around the eyes (for brows), mouth, and lip at the same time as removing the hair. It is obviously not as messy as waxing. And unlike waxing, you can have threading done on stubble (roughly two days after shaving is ideal).

WAXING

Waxing entails applying hot wax to your hair and pressing paper or cloth into it. When the wax sets, you rip it off quickly, pulling off the hair with the wax. It can be as painful as it sounds, especially for large areas. Many people report the pain as excruciating, especially in sensitive areas. Others say it doesn't hurt much or they get used to it over time. Try a small area first and see how you can tolerate the pain, before getting your legs waxed. Your hair inevitably grows back sooner than you hope, so make sure the pain and money are worth it. The rate your hair grows back depends on your genes, not on the waxing or technique; therefore, if one friend reports it takes a whole week, it is due to her hair growth rate, not waxing.

Like tweezing, waxing stimulates the roots and hair follicles. You can get lucky sometimes and create scar tissue in the follicle, inhibiting hair growth, although this usually doesn't happen. Ingrown hairs are a common side effect, and waxing can cause skin irritation. Many women wax for years without any problems, and find this method satisfying, especially for facial hair. Trimming long hair with scissors first makes waxing easier.

Cost and Convenience

Wax can be purchased in pots at major retail stores and specialty stores that cater to salon products. Waxes vary in quality and effectiveness, so you might want to ask for advice or check consumer guides before purchasing a particular brand.

Basic at-home wax treatments cost between $5 and $20 and require special heating instructions and great care when self-waxing. Heating the wax in a microwave oven instead of a stovetop can result in uneven heating and serious burns. Waxing is messy and takes time, but is quicker than a trip to a salon. Waxing becomes easier with practice.

Some manufacturers make wax strips that are good for upper lip hair removal for women on the go. These strips are inexpensive (about $8 for a package of twenty strips) and do not require preheating.

Waxing is readily available through most salons for the upper lip and eyebrow. A session costs about $8 for the upper lip, although some salons charge up to $30. Some women will go to salons for years to do larger areas, thinking that it is cheaper than other methods. However, over time the cost and time commitment adds up. It is worth comparing waxing with electrolysis and laser therapy.

Unwanted Hair and Hirsutism

Use extreme caution at salons, as thousands of women have been injured. Read page 103 to learn tips on how to avoid dangerous waxing experiences. Some states license or certify professional waxers.

HOME ELECTROLYSIS KITS

Home electrolysis kits deserve some mention, as many women have them in their closet. They usually involve a DC battery, which powers a fine wire filament that conducts electricity into the hair follicle. The good news is that the battery isn't strong enough to do a lot of damage to the skin; the bad news is that there is no way the layperson can know how to properly insert the filament into the follicle (at what depth, angle, etc.). As a result, the hair is actually tweezed out instead of being removed via electrolysis, and therefore is not permanently removed.

Even a trained professional would be hard pressed to perform electrolysis on her own face because of magnification requirements (a mirror can only present a backward image), though some flexible individuals can and do perform electrolysis on other parts of their own body. Most home electrolysis kits are available through mail order for $10 to $200.

If you are considering a purchase to save money, consider the following:

- It takes an enormous amount of time to learn and execute.
- It is painful.
- It is not recommended to use on your face because of having to use a mirror, and then moving your hand in an opposite direction. If you doubt this advice, try drawing a pattern on your face using a mirror (use a lipstick liner or something else you can wipe away).
- If you don't use this device properly, it is not a permanent solution. So why not use something easier and more reliable?

If you're lured into buying a home electrolysis kit through the Internet, home shopping channels, or other vehicles, contact the American Electrology Association to discuss the item you want to purchase. Also check consumer guides to verify reviews and look for scams.

MISCELLANEOUS HAIR REMOVAL PRODUCTS AND SCAMS

Clearly, there are so many products available because people are buying them. Even brand-name companies are marketing products that don't work. Virtually every woman does some kind of hair removal or has in the past, or will in the future, making these products and services big business.

Scammers have figured out women's vulnerability and are capitalizing on it. The Internet has opened up many more opportunities for con artists to get your money. Chat rooms are filled with women complaining about various products, and the FDA has made some illegal for use on certain areas of the body.

If you don't see a hair removal method discussed in this book, be particularly cautious. If the FDA approves of a new product after this book is published, you will hear about it from legitimate independent sources, not some proprietary Web site.

For an overview of scams, see HairFacts at www.hairfacts.com. The publishers do a nice job of researching and listing fraudulent brands and the con artists who make them. They have even exposed a pornographer selling a topical cream under the brands Ultra Hair Away and Victoria Bodyworks. He seems to have made a smart marketing move by using names that can be searched on the Internet by people trying to find Victoria's Secret and the Body Shop. These scams are not just about taking your money, they are products that can hurt your skin and cause pain. Hairfacts.com cautions against all products sold on television. The site also exposes companies that falsely claim to have FDA approval.

Here is an easy way to detect a fraud: Electrolysis is the only method of permanent hair removal (however, beware of home electrolysis kits). Conductive gels, patches, microwaves, and so forth that claim to work "just like electrolysis without the needles" are scams, too. It is impossible for them to work for the same reason that the tweezers-type devices cannot work: hair is not a conductor of electricity. For more information, contact the American Electrology Association.

SUMMARY OF ELECTROLYSIS AND LASER TREATMENT

Electrolysis and laser treatment are so effective and popular that this book devotes an entire chapter to each method of hair removal. See chapters 9 and 10 for a discussion on the pros and cons and make informed decisions.

For either treatment, hair will continue to grow unless you address any underlying hormonal problem. Consult an endocrinologist if you have an excessive amount of hair, new hair growth, or if you have hair growing in a typical male pattern (see figure 3 in chapter 3).

Electrolysis will permanently remove hair that is already there, but if your body is producing too much androgen, new hairs will continue to be converted to terminal hairs, making electrolysis a never-ending process.

Electrolysis versus Laser Treatment

Laser hair removal is gaining popularity, but its success depends on your hair and skin pigment. The less pigment in your hair, the less effective the laser treatment is because the laser can't grasp the pigment in the hair, which is how it works. Conversely, the more pigment in the skin, the more difficult it is to administer because the laser attaches to the pigment in the skin as well as to the hair. *Laser removal is most effective if you are fair-skinned and dark-haired.* If you are removing light hair that has less pigment, electrolysis works but laser does not.

Electrolysis cuts across race and works equally well for women of all skin shades and of all hair textures and colors. Electrolysis is less expensive than laser treatment for small areas. Because it is permanent, over many years electrolysis is less expensive for all areas; however, laser is considered easier and better for large areas of hair because electrolysis works hair by hair, taking more time for large areas.

Laser is also considered less painful and more comfortable than electrolysis. Anecdotally, males experience more pain from laser than women (maybe women are just used to hair-plucking pain!). For both procedures, some parts of the body are more painful than others.

If your hair and skin meet the criteria for effective laser treatment, and you hire a trained technician who used the correct laser device for your hair and skin, there is no real evidence that electrolysis or laser is better. It depends on your goals and your tolerance for regrowth and pain. This lack of definitiveness is because the two methods have not been studied and compared as of this writing only cursory scientific trials that have not yielded much information.

There is no reason you can't use both laser and electrolysis. You may not be able to have them at the same time, but certainly you can use them as you need or want. There are some technicians and clinics that offer both electrolysis and laser. If you are interested in both, or are not sure about which technique is best, consult with a technician or a clinic how to best treat your problem areas.

CHAPTER 8

HAIR REMOVAL BY BODY PART

EYEBROW SHAPING

In high school I tweezed the stray hairs between my eyebrows. When my daughters looked at some old pictures of me they noticed that I removed too many hairs between my eyebrows. I agreed and we laughed about it. Now in my forties, I have one hair that grows out of a mole on my face and when I think about it I cut it with scissors. I have been thinking lately that I should have it permanently removed somehow, but have not really looked into it. I might even remove the entire mole because it has become raised and it annoys me. Cosmetically, I don't know which would look worse—a mole or a scar. I'm sure I will have more hair issues as I age.

People in my family are not very hairy. In fact, my mother needs to paint eyebrows on because she hardly has any hair. I want to be careful not to over pluck my eyebrows because I think if you fool with them too much, you end up not having any as you age. I probably walk around with bushy eyebrows, but I like them and no one else has ever commented to me that I should change them. —N.D.

If you don't like your eyebrows the way they are, it is a good idea to have your first tweezing or waxing done by a competent relative, friend, or a professional. Another good reason to treat them well is because out of all our hair, eyebrow follicles are the most sensitive to injury. Just one or two plucks could damage the hair irreversibly and it won't grow back.

Carefully think through shaping your eyebrows. Do you really want to change the shape of your eyebrows, and how? Do you just want to remove the connector between your eyebrows, or really shape them differently?

And please consider very thoroughly any idea to remove them all and pencil them back in. There is absolutely no way to recreate hair with a pencil on your face, and think about all the hassle involved in redrawing them everyday! Not to mention you might look cartoonish.

Another reason to be cautious with your eyebrow shaping is because there are a lot of different standards about how eyebrows should look, and the fashion changes periodically. If you don't like the shapes now, try again next year. When Brooke Shields became popular, just think of all the women with plucked-skinny eyebrows kicking themselves.

Remember these points as well: Your eyebrows are on your face for a reason. They protect your eyes. They naturally reflect your bone structure, therefore imposing an eyebrow shape from someone ethnically different than you onto your face will not look the same as the woman in the magazine.

Look for a shape that flatters your face, just as you do your haircut. Do you want a hairstyle you have to style every day? If the answer is no, you may have the same answer about your eyebrows. Just like different hair growth rates on heads, your eyebrows might grow in faster than another woman's.

Eyebrow Plucking Warning

Eyebrows are easy targets for twitchy fingers. We see our face throughout the day in the bathroom, we hold our head in our hands, we scratch our itches, and we see hair pop up that no one else does.

The problem is that if you pull the hair on the edge of your eyebrows or over the bridge of your nose, as it reacts and becomes stronger and coarser it does not lie down and behave as it once did. Hair may even grow back pointing in the opposite direction! The best alternative is to make a plan for professional shaping or keep your impulsive fingers at bay.

Eyebrow Waxing at Nail Salons

There seems to be a nail salon on every corner—and they usually offer eyebrow waxing. Not only are there many of these storefronts, but many are ripe with infection. Many states regulate the nail stores, but many do not. For instance, many states are strict about cutting nail cuticles, and others have no rules or don't enforce them. Some states regulate waxing technicians, many do not.

Get referrals and look for certificates from the government on the wall. Legally, government certificates must be posted prominently and a good store wants you to see its certificates. Research if your state is one behind the times in terms of regulating these nail stores. If it is, you should be extra cautious about cleanliness and experience. Generally, states with little business regulation and higher concentrations of poverty, occupational accidents, and disease rates—the southern U.S. states—have the least amount of consumer protections. (New York and Washington don't license electrologists at the time of this writing, either.)

Countless women have gotten an infection or severe pain from bad waxing techniques and unsterile conditions. If you have any suspicions, leave the salon immediately. Here are a few things to look for:

- The technician should put on a new pair of gloves in your sight.
- The waxing table should have clean paper covering it.
- The technician should show you the sterilizing solution and tools.
- If you are having your pubic or bikini area waxed, you should be offered disposable underwear.

Besides risking infection, if you go to a nail place without a real professional, they will tell you exactly what you want to hear without understanding your hair type or shape of your face, or asking about your goals. Ask questions that don't require a yes or no answer, to make sure you are not being "yesed." If you go along with a persuasive salesperson who is not competent, you risk receiving a shape that is different than your natural brow bone and hair pattern; you then must battle to maintain the shape or to prevent the stubs from growing in and looking like you have two layers of eyebrows. Remember, repeated waxing or tweezing generally makes the hair grow in stronger, coarser, and darker.

A professional will show you examples and understand your needs. Will you be coming back weekly? Will you "clean it up" yourself, and if so, how often? Make sure the professional understands the amount (density) of your eyebrows, texture, and growth rate. Check out her clientele, too. If she is not used to shaping thick eyebrows such as yours, she may not be the right person for you.

Unfortunately, shaping your eyebrows is not like getting a bad haircut that grows in. Yes, your eyebrows will grow in to their natural shape, but only after you let the stubs grow out. In the beginning phases of eyebrow shaping you may not have stubbly eyebrow hair, yet, and it will still be fine and lie down while it grows back. But over time this will change.

Here are some questions to ask yourself before you get ready to shape your eyebrows:

Unwanted Hair and Hirsutism

- How much deviation do you want from your natural line?
- How many times a week or month do you want to maintain the shape?
- Which shapes match your hair texture?
- How frequently do you want to return to a professional, if at all?

The irony, of course, is that eyebrow hair is one of the areas that stops growing as we age. So, while you may be unhappy about your eyebrows now, when you approach your forties, you will see them lessen, and then perhaps one day you will wonder where your bounteous hair has gone. Of all our hair, eyebrows and eyelashes have the shortest regrowth life. Your eyebrow hair will naturally fall out, but they won't all grow back in.

Cost and Convenience

Eyebrow shaping—usually by waxing—is becoming increasingly convenient. As mentioned previously, there are many storefront shops for quick waxing. As threading becomes more popular, you may have even more options.

The cost varies widely. You may want to spring for the big-bucks treatment, $35 or more, a few times a year, and do the in-between times yourself with a good pair of tweezers, or go to a reputable, clean, and competent storefront for $8 a pop.

If you want or need a professional's help more frequently, see if you can negotiate a "customer loyalty" discount. Someone who gets to know you and may have some time in her schedule when she is less busy than others may be willing to give you a discount, or at least the fifth time free.

If you are really struggling with your eyebrows, consider electrolysis. It is permanent, so the investment might be worth it if you have a lot of hair to cope with. Because it is permanent, consider the minimal amount of removal for the following reasons:

1. Hair fashions for eyebrows change and you don't want to be stuck with an outdated style.
2. As you age, you will lose eyebrow hair and thin eyebrows will look even thinner.
3. You may become more accepting of your hair over time and regret taking too much off and deviating from what you were born with.

NOSE AND EAR HAIR

> *There comes a time in every man's life when his body goes through changes. The boy transforms into man. And then many years later, when he feels on top of his game, Mother Nature comes out of nowhere to blindside him once again. It is a time of wonder, discovery, and awkward freakishness. The most obvious change is the arrival of ear and nose hair. This can suck.*
> —www.shaveeverywhere.com

The Philips Norelco Web site (www.consumer.phillips.com) has found a way to entice men to buy their razors and grooming kits. They use a humorous video with the main character shocked at a nose hair that just keeps growing and growing. Then the dad gives his grown son a cartoon pamphlet like you'd get in school to describe puberty, which they call second puberty. It is true, just when you are feeling competent and mature, strange hairs pop up—for everyone, not just men.

Nose hair is another area twitchy fingers can't resist. You probably notice more hair growing out of your nose as you age. Nose hair filters germs and keeps your nostrils—and therefore your respiratory system—healthy, so definitely don't remove them from the follicles, just clip them so they are not popping out of your nose. If you are tempted to pull or tweeze, remember that those hairs will just come in darker, coarser, and in strange angles, causing you more angst.

Also, plucking hair from the tender nostril tissues can result easily in soreness or an infection. Nose hair clippers or nose hair trimmers are made to trim this hair and keep it out of the way of tissues and your mucus. Unfortunately, since their target audience is men, the clippers in the local drugstores are rather large for most women and scary to use. Try a department store in the women's section or shop online for something suitable.

"A nose hair clipper is a personal grooming device used to trim excess hair in the nostrils and ears," according to www.wisegeek.com. This is how a nose hair clipper's technology and use is explained on its Web site:

> Most nose hair clipper devices use a set of small rotary blades protected by a chrome or stainless steel housing. A battery-powered electric motor is used to turn these blades, and external combs protect the skin from contacting the blades directly. Individual

hairs are guided into the cutting zone and safely trimmed off. A quality nose hair clipper can usually be rinsed under water while in use. The entire device can often be immersed for thorough cleaning and sanitizing between uses.

The basic technique for trimming unwanted ear and nose hair is to activate the nose hair clipper and carefully insert it into the proper canal. As individual hairs enter the cutting chamber, sharp rotary blades slice through them cleanly. Some nostril hair is necessary for protection against dust and germs, so the user shouldn't aim for complete nasal baldness.

A nose hair clipper can also be used to remove excessive ear hair from the external canal area. A mirror should be used to guide the clipper to the right spots. There are also manual clipper models, which act like nail clippers; they are a little harder to find than electronic ones. You can use safety scissors to cut your hair (the kind with the round edge) as well.

Cost and Convenience
The cost ranges from $10 to $100 for clippers. Opt for quality, as some models go through their batteries fast. Dying batteries are an ongoing expense, but also the clipper might start yanking rather than clean-cutting your hair as the battery dies, which can hurt and harm your nostril. Do not wait it out; replace the batteries at the first sign of warning.

You can bring trimmers on trips, tuck one away in your closet, or put one in your briefcase, making them very convenient. The manual ones are even more convenient because you don't need batteries and can tuck them in your purse for a quick clip in the restroom.

TOES, BELLY BUTTON/HAPPY TRAIL, FINGERS
Hair in these areas generally does not grow very densely. As discussed, tweezing them will make them stronger, longer, and darker. It is also extremely likely no one but you notices hair on your toes or fingers. Small, sharp scissors that you can get close to your skin is the best option for some of these areas, electronic trimmers may work for others, and bleaching or waxing is appropriate for other areas, depending on your preference. A word of caution: Using methods that foster hair growth and thicker strands can make these hair types look bushy, therefore avoid yanking from the follicle.

Unwanted Hair and Hirsutism

Natural bleaching works, too. Chances are, if you are reading this book, you have dark-pigmented skin, so a little sun won't burn you. Get outside and walk on the beach, garden, or walk in sandals and expose your body to sunlight. The sunlight will naturally lighten your hair to a shade that likely blends well with your skin. Hair that is removed won't have a chance to lighten on its own. If you have been indoors all winter and are just noticing dark hair, don't worry; it doesn't take long for the sun to do its job. The vitamin D your body absorbs is also very important for your bones.

BIKINI AREA AND INNER THIGHS

It has become culturally fashionable—if not expected in some circles—to remain hairless right up to the line of one's bathing suit or panties. Prior to the days when waxing or sugaring was popular in North America, women often just shaved these areas. If you look at the bathing suits of yesteryear (e.g., 1940s through early 1960s), the panty line was much more generous than it is today. This has all changed, of course. Some women feel mortified if a stray hair pops out, as if we don't all have pubic hair. Women's shaving margins have widened, just as the bikini margin has narrowed.

There are more choices in bathing suit bottoms these days than there were thirty years ago, so you can choose a wider one or one with a skirt. Trimming the edge of your pubic hair with a pair of scissors or using another method will prevent the dark hairs from sticking out. Trimming the inside of the thighs also may be enough for you to avoid the social stigma you may feel. If you don't feel comfortable with your hair and are not vacationing in Europe, then most methods work, albeit with some irritation or tenderness. Ingrown hairs in the bikini area are especially painful as they rub against a snug bathing suit or underwear.

If you want to shave to your bikini line, you can do it yourself in the shower with a good moisturizing shaving cream. Try wearing your bathing suit in the shower to get a good "fit." For aftercare, use gel from an aloe plant (be sure to buy pure aloe or an aloe plant to avoid perfumes and other irritating chemicals).

Hair removal cream works well, too. If you are doing the whole leg, put the cream on the inside of your thighs up to the bikini line last to avoid burning.

Unwanted Hair and Hirsutism

There are bikini-waxing kits available for home use, but you must be careful to follow the directions exactly. The waxes used for bikini and pubic areas are gentler than what is generally sold for upper lip waxing. If you choose a salon to do it for you, they often use talcum powders in combination with the wax to minimize irritation. It is especially important you choose a safe place that you trust for bikini-area waxing. You definitely don't want to get an infection there.

Some new products on the market are bikini kits that contain electronic, waterproof trimmers and aftercare cream. These do-it-yourself spa treatments are nothing more than trimmers and high-end packaging for razors. They are much more expensive than buying a trimmer and aloe separately and have questionable results. Be sure to look for consumer ratings before you buy.

If you go to a spa for any of these methods, please read the information about sanitation and licensing on page 149.

FACE

> *Even though laser treatment for my facial hair was painful—especially the first time!—I have only had to go twice in the last two years. I used to go for waxing or threading at least every other month or bleach my facial hair. I hated how waxing made my face red and I started noticing wrinkles.* —H.A.

Facial skin is sensitive. Across-the-board epilation and most other types of hair removal is painful, yet shaving facial hair is stigmatizing and makes women feel as though they are abnormal. Even though millions of women tweeze and wax their face, it is not considered acceptable for women to shave their face because of the resulting stubble. The problem with shaving for women is where on their body stubble is socially and culturally acceptable. Shaving legs and underarms and revealing stubble in these areas is the norm.

In light of this, medical specialists recommend that women refrain from shaving the face if it does not feel comfortable, but they do not discourage shaving if the woman's goal is to remove the hair without stimulating the roots.

If your goal is to permanently remove facial hair, shaving or cutting, of course, will not do this, but it is a better alternative for some parts or quantities than waxing, tweezing, or sugaring. Be warned, however, once you begin shaving on a regular basis, you may have a constant battle with stubble and therefore may want to consider electrolysis. If you opt to shave a facial area, use an electric razor.

Cutting facial hair with scissors or a trimmer is a good alternative, depending on how much hair you want to get rid of. Tweezers can also do the job on a chin hair or two that bothers you, as long as you know the ramifications. Be careful when you use magnifying mirrors; you may see hair that you and others would not have noticed. You probably do not want to look like the witch on a broomstick with hair coming out of a mole, but you don't need to go overboard taking any hair you see out, especially with tweezers.

If you have a lot of hair and bleach is not a viable option, electrolysis on some of the follicles or laser treatment may reduce it enough to lessen your self-consciousness and in the end may be cheaper than repeated waxing or threading. Waxing and threading are popular temporary methods; however, after many years, you may find you have to maintain the method you choose as the hair grows back stronger and possibly thicker.

NECK, BACK, AND TORSO

> *When we were kids, my sister and I thought it was hilarious that my mother would arbitrarily choose the spots where my Dad's neck started and ended. He was so furry that the hair on his head merged with the hair on his neck and down his back. My mom would just choose a place to start shaving at the bottom of his head and shave it down to the spot where she determined his shoulders began.*
>
> *My brother did not find this so funny, maybe because he knew he was looking at his future. I didn't know I was looking at my future, too. But when I have short haircuts the hairdresser shaves the hair that grows down my neck, far below most women's hairline.*
>
> *A couple of months ago I was getting ready to go to a wedding. It was a few weeks after a haircut and my husband said, "Uh, before we go, I'd better shave your neck." He does it every few weeks between haircuts. It probably needs to be done more, but we both forget. Luckily, he doesn't mind a slightly scruffy wife.*
>
> *My hairiness, neck and otherwise, has not been a source of discomfort. I like it. Most of the time. There are some parts that are not so endearing to me, like the weird, dark long strays on my face that started when I was in my forties. That's too scruffy for me.* —P.A.

Unwanted Hair and Hirsutism

Shaving your neck and back can be dangerous if not downright impossible to do by yourself. These areas may require a supportive partner, family member, or professional's help. If you want to remove this hair, think of it as part of your regimen, like dying your hair every few months, clipping your nails, or washing your delicate clothes. Once it becomes part of your routine it will fit normally into your life and perhaps any self-consciousness will dissipate.

Try a men's electric razor. They are cheaper than women's razors and give a closer shave. If the hair is sparse or the area is limited, scissors (made for hair cutting) might do the job well and won't leave you with razor stubble.

CHAPTER 9

REMOVING PUBIC HAIR

It's just plain creepy. Why do so many men want to have sex with a partner that looks like a prepubescent girl? I don't mind trimming my hair back so it stays out of the way while peeing or during sex, but removing it? How is being childlike sexy? I don't want any man treating me like a child. Besides, with the rate my hair grows, my skin only will feel smooth for a day. — M.M.

It may be inaccurate to categorize pubic hair as "unwanted" in that it is necessary body hair, but women are now being influenced by the media and their partners to shape and groom their pubic hair to make their genitals supposedly more attractive. Popular television programs such as *Sex and the City* have helped to advance its cause by sending their characters for Brazilian bikini waxes—the "female circumcision" of bikini waxes, which leaves only a small patch of hair over the clitoris. A Brazilian wax is far from a bikini wax—and the bikini line. Not to be outdone by the Brazilians, in the United States shaping or fully removing all pubic hair is now fashionable. Perhaps it is related to a shift in sexual behaviors and the increase in oral sex for people looking for safe alternatives to intercourse to reduce their risks of contracting sexually transmitted diseases.

Some men—and women—like the hairless sensation during sex. For some, their hair is fine in texture and does not hurt as it grows back. This only works if the man is clean-cut, too; otherwise, his coarse pubic hair can irritate you. Some women like the way their hairless body looks. If you use a temporary method lsuch as shaving or waxing, you can easily grow your pubic hair back when the fashion changes.

There is, however, a distressing trend of sexualizing girls in our culture—in effect comparing adult woman, who are fully sexual beings, to preadolescents. Pubic hair only comes with maturity, so to consider an adult woman's genitals now less sexual than that of a girl's is insulting. And worse, finding a girl's body sexually stimulating is generally considered the terrain of perverts. It's shocking to find this sexualization of girls in the mainstream. (There are books and studies being done about marketing sex both to girls and to would-be perverts, if you want to read up on it.)

You can resist these media messages by questioning just what your definition of maturity is. Take pride in being a woman, both in mind and body. You probably fought long and hard to be taken seriously as an adult, so don't give it up now for what is probably a passing trend. Promoting women to appear like girls appeals to many men. For them it's dominance, the ideal of "deflowering" a virgin, or perhaps they are insecure with their own manhood and therefore want to be in control of someone they feel is young and vulnerable. Even men who aren't so insecure can be influenced easily by popular culture, especially as it hits the mainstream and is seemingly normal.

If your partner brings up removing your pubic hair, even in jest, remember he may be exploring your opinion and is not so set on it himself. After all, he has pubic hair, too. Talk to him about cultural norms and about seeing you as a woman and not a girl. If your partner thinks you are prudish or unadventurous, or if you are trying to withstand his pressure, then ask him to remove his pubic hair first. If he's not willing, well, then you may have an uneven relationship. Whatever you choose to do, make sure it is your reason and one you embrace. Peer pressure stories from friends or in magazines may not detail the horrible itching while the hair grows back in, or describe the grooming needed in addition to shaving your legs or other areas. Articles promoting removing pubic hair seldom describe the infections one is prone to, either. And like any peer pressure, most of the people doing it are all talk. Also, consider that as you age, your pubic hair will not replenish and you'll have less of it (so tell your partner to wait).

If you are curious about what you look like bald, try a close scissor cut first. To read more about this topic, read *Body Drama* (Redd 2008), a book for young women that covers many nonmedical hair topics. If you prefer the feeling or look of being hairless or want to try it, first consider the following benefits of pubic hair before removing it.

BENEFITS OF PUBIC HAIR

Pubic hair is thicker than normal body hair and has a sheen to it. Its purpose is to protect the *vulva*, the external part of your genitals. Although many people think the vulva is one of the many outer genitals, such as the vaginal lips, the vulva is simply a general term that refers to a whole collection of parts. In the same way that your face refers to a collection of parts like your eyes, nose, and mouth, your vulva is the "face" of the genitals.

Unwanted Hair and Hirsutism

Your vulva consists of the following parts:

- Mons, the area above your genitals covered with pubic hair
- Clitoris, a sexual organ made of erectile tissue that, when stimulated, leads to orgasm
- Urinary opening
- Outer and inner lips of the vagina
- Vaginal opening
- Perineum, the area of skin that separates your anus from your vagina
- Anus

Your pubic hair acts as a necessary safety net, protecting your vulva from infections and irritations by blocking what can get in and onto the parts of your vulva, including dangerous bacteria that can cause infections. If you remove your pubic hair, you are more vulnerable to bacterial infections. If you've ever had a urinary tract infection, you know how painful and inconvenient they are.

WHICH METHOD IS BEST?

One good thing about getting old, you get less pubic and underarm hair to deal with. Makes a trip to the beach a lot easier. —A.S.

Pubic hair is a necessary part of your anatomy, so use only a temporary hair removal method such as shaving or waxing so your hair can grow back. You may want your public hair back some day if you become pregnant or change your attitude about what you find attractive. And when you become postmenopausal and lose your hair, you want it back and kick yourself over something you did in your younger years. It is not like a tattoo that you can get removed.

Some women use hair removal creams in this area, but this is highly discouraged because of the harsh chemicals in these creams. They can badly irritate the delicate skin of the vulva, and get into your vagina, causing irritations of nightmarish proportion.

Do not use electrolysis or laser treatment in this delicate area, either. A professional waxing is the best method. The technician—hopefully certified and experienced—should be adept. If you want a Brazilian wax, find someone who knows what they are and what they are supposed to look like; don't assume any nail salon can perform one. The best way to find one is to ask other women who are satisfied clients.

To remove hair around the anus and perineum, do so very carefully! Do not shave it or use any electronic device that can slice this very delicate skin, or hot wax or sugar that can tear the skin. Pull the hair away from your skin and use scissors but avoid a close cut. If you use a mirror, be sure to practice first mastering the reverse direction your hand will seem to move. If you tweeze, do only a few hairs at a time to avoid inflammation and infection.

Hygiene Precautions for Brazilian Waxing

Here are some hygiene rules to follow if you decide to go "Brazilian" or even further:

- Do not use products with chemicals or perfumes in that area. Even shampoos and conditioners can irritate the delicate skin if you are rinsing your hair in the shower.
- Keep the area well moisturized.
- Use unscented sanitary napkins and change them frequently or use cotton sanitary pads. Cotton pads are far more comfortable than paper pads and they are washable, which saves you tons of money and our world lots of trees. Try vendors such as GladRags and Êma Pads, which make products friendly to women's bodies. They are available online, in health food stores, co-ops and other eco-friendly stores.
- Get some lavender essential oil and add a few drops to a bath each night, or use mild or natural lotions made with the oil. Lavender will help to soothe and heal the area. Herbalists claim that it balances the hormone system and is good for the female reproductive system.

HOW TO AVOID VAGINAL INFECTIONS

Vulvitis

One of the most common problems associated with removing pubic hair is being predisposed to *vulvitis*, which means "inflammation of the vulva," characterized by an itchy, red, swollen vulva and, in extreme cases, even blistering. Diabetic women are particularly vulnerable to vulvitis because of certain complications of the disease. Postmenopausal women can develop vulvitis because their tissue in this area becomes less elastic, thinner, drier, and more susceptible to irritation. Scratching only makes it worse.

A number of factors cause vulvitis, including external irritants such as fabric allergies (e.g., latex, which is commonly found in many underwear brands), powders, soaps, colored toilet tissue, and perfumes. Oral sex can also trigger vulvitis, as can sanitary napkins, medications, diet, stress, or sexually transmitted diseases and other infections (e.g., yeast infections).

The best way to deal with vulvitis is to isolate the cause first, especially if it is an allergy or a bacterial infection. Or if you frequently get vulvitis because of menopause or diabetes, avoid cleaning your vulva with soap (which can be an irritant), and consult a dermatologist for advice.

Treat your vulva as you would your face: keep it moisturized. The extra lubrication really helps prevent irritation and vulvitis. You can see how just the process of removing your public hair can be irritating to your vulva, let alone the resulting exposure to sun, air, water, and other drying and irritating elements, so keep it lubricated and protected from dirty clothes, sheets, and people.

Yeast Infections

Here are some good rules to follow if you suffer from yeast infections:

- Do not wear tight clothing around your vagina. Tight pants, panties, and pantyhose may prevent your vagina from breathing and make it warmer and moister for yeast. Switch to knee-highs, thigh-highs, or old-fashioned stockings, or limit your pantyhose wearing for special occasions.
- Go "bottomless" to bed to let air into your vagina.
- Wear only 100 percent cotton clothing and/or natural fibers around your vagina. Synthetic (e.g., nylon) underwear and polyester pants are not good ideas. All cotton underwear and loose-fitting denim, silk, or rayon pants are fine. If you must wear pantyhose without underwear, make sure you wear the kind with a cotton lining.
- Change your sanitary pads frequently or wear cotton ones.

- Do not use vaginal deodorants or sprays. These are unnecessary and disturb the vagina's natural environment, which is fully designed to self-clean.
- Do not douche unless it is recommended by your physician. Douching can push harmful bacteria higher into the vagina, disturb the vagina's natural ecosystem, or interfere with a pregnancy.
- Watch your toilet habits. Always wipe from front to back. Otherwise, you can introduce rectal material and germs into your vagina. After a loose bowel movement, wet the toilet paper and clean your rectal area so that fecal material doesn't stay on your underwear and wind up in your vagina.
- Don't insert anything into a dry vagina. Whether it is a penis or a tampon, make sure your vagina is well lubricated before insertion. Dry vaginas can be scraped during insertion, which can lead to infection.
- Avoid wearing tampons. If you must wear tampons, limit the amount of time they stay in, change them every two or three hours, and do not wear them to bed. Try organic cotton tampons from such companies as NatraCare and Organic Essentials.

WOMEN WHO SHOULD NOT REMOVE THEIR PUBIC HAIR

If any of the following statements are true, you should not have a Brazilian wax or remove significant amounts of your pubic hair.

- *I have diabetes.* Removing too much pubic hair can cause repeated infections.
- *I am in perimenopause.* Removing pubic hair can worsen the discomforts of perimenopause.
- *I am postmenopausal.* Dryness worsens without pubic hair.
- *I suffer from repeated yeast infections.* Removing pubic hair can exacerbate yeast infections.
- *I have a sexually transmitted disease.* Removing pubic hair can exacerbate any STD.
- *I am pregnant.* Pubic hair protects harmful bacteria from entering the cervix.

Unwanted Hair and Hirsutism

- *I have had a gynecological procedure done within the last three months.* You may still be healing and need your pubic hair for protection.
- *I am taking antibiotics.* You are more susceptible to vaginal infections during this time; keep your pubic hair for now.
- *I am taking drugs that suppress my immune system.* Again, you are more susceptible to vaginal infections during this time; keep your pubic hair for now.
- *I have skin allergies.* If you are prone to rashes or have chronic skin allergies, keep your pubic hair.
- *I have eczema.* You know how itchy and painful that can be on your hand, multiply that on the sensitive pubic area.

CHAPTER 10

ELECTROLYSIS: WHAT YOU NEED TO KNOW

> *I see a lot of older women who spent many years taking care of their children. Many come in habitually covering their mouth and chin. I see their self-esteem and confidence rise after treatment, especially women with hormone disorders. Many of my clients feel as if they're the only ones with a problem. I dispel that notion and work on the most important areas to them first. Many cry with relief and I receive gifts and letters from happy customers.* —Patsy Kirby, MA, CPE, former executive director of the American Electrology Association

Electrolysis is currently the only way to permanently remove hair. If you have the time to spare, and can afford it, electrolysis can be used on just about all areas of your body. Electrolysis also treats ingrown hairs and folliculitis.

The method is foolproof; however, depending on the coarseness of the hair and its growth cycle, a series of treatments may be required to permanently disable a follicle. If you are going to have electrolysis treatment for hair on your face, breasts, or other delicate areas, shaving before electrolysis removes the hair just "hanging out," waiting to shed. Only actively growing hair strands rise through the surface of the skin, which is what you want because electrolysis destroys hair in the anagen (growth) phase. Electrolysis can remove hairs in the catagen (transition) and telogen (resting) phases; however, there is little or no destruction during these stages, and the hair from these follicles grows back.

A technician called an *electrologist* uses a very fine needle, placing it alongside the hair shaft and into the hair follicle. The needle is about the size of a hair itself. It is not an injection; electrolysis is akin to tattooing except that the needle is solid, not hollow. A mild electric current is delivered via the needle to destroy the hair growth cells (dermal papilla among others) at the bottom of the follicle, thereby disabling regeneration.

Unwanted Hair and Hirsutism

Figure 6. Electrolysis Probe in Hair Follicle

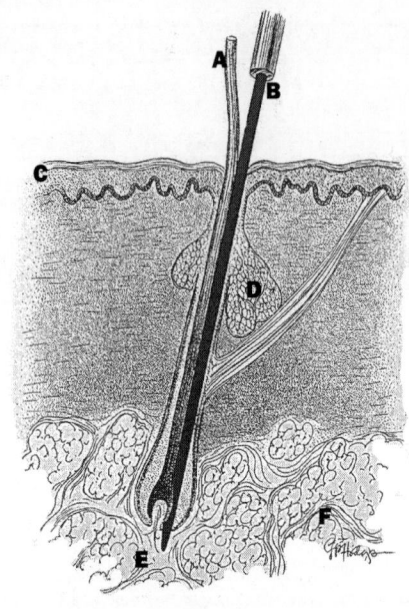

A. Hair shaft
B. Probe
C. Layers of skin
D. Oil gland
E. Capillaries
F. Dermal papilla vein

Photomicrographs and many more are available from Prestige Electrolysis Supply, 1-800-783-7403, www.prestigeelec.com.

The biggest problem with electrolysis is the misinformation circulating around it. The information in this chapter helps dispel some common myths. Electrolysis is said to be very painful and prohibitively expensive; it is neither, if done correctly. Another common misconception is that you need only one treatment per hair.

Electrolysis should be done by a skilled and certified technician. Any time something pierces your skin, you should take the utmost care to protect yourself, including checking the technician's credentials. The authority on electrolysis in the United States is the American Electrology Association (AEA), recognized by the Centers for Disease Control and Prevention (CDC) and the Food and Drug Administration (FDA) as the authoritative source for information about unwanted hair and its safe, permanent removal. For more information, contact the AEA or visit its Web site at www.electrology.com.

Before delving into the details of myths and safety precautions, take a look at the how electrolysis works and how it developed into a treatment you now find at salons and spas.

A BRIEF HISTORY OF ELECTROLYSIS

Electrolysis was first developed in 1875 by Dr. Charles E. Michel, an eye surgeon in Missouri who used it to remove ingrown eyelashes. The method began to take off in the late 1890s. By 1916, Paul N. Kree developed the "multiple needle technique" for galvanic electrolysis, basically a chemical process. Galvanic treatment is what we have today. It is not actually the electric current itself, but the chemical reaction our body has to it that destroys the hair growth cells.

When a needle is introduced into the hair follicle and the current is applied, the body's salt and water (i.e., moisture in the tissues) react, rearranging themselves into three constituent chemical elements: sodium hydroxide (lye), hydrogen gas, and chlorine gas. This process is called *electrolysis*. The gases are of little concern to the electrologist, but the lye, being highly caustic, is an effective instrument of destruction when produced in the tiny hair follicle. Simply put, the lye is what attacks the tissue, not the current.

Over time, electrolysis began to spread into the hands of lay professionals instead of being offered only by physicians. In the early 1920s a newer method was developed in France, called *thermolysis* (also short-wave, diathermy, high-frequency, or "flash"), which proved to be faster.

Flash thermolysis is a brief heat source delivered via the needle. It acts by cauterizing or electro-desiccating (drying up) the regenerative cells. If the needle is not on target, however, there will be less destruction to the hair growth cells than with the blend (another method invented in the 1940s) or galvanic method alone. There are no medical studies proving that "blending" galvanic electrolysis and thermolysis is more effective than using one or the other; however, many practitioners believe that it is.

For example, if insufficient current is applied with short-wave thermolysis, you will have to keep destroying the regenerative cells. The possibility of applying insufficient current is more likely with heavy, coarse hair—the ones you likely want to get rid of. Fine, vellus hair tends to respond quite well to thermolysis.

Unwanted Hair and Hirsutism

Those with coarse hair might look into *manual thermolysis*, a variation on this technique, which uses less intensity with longer timing than the flash techniques. Any method utilizing galvanic current, as well as some epilators using an automatic thermolysis technique, requires that the patient hold a "ground" or what is called an indifferent or positive electrode. An electrologist will often use a disposable moist wrap, cloth, or a conduction cream for better conductivity.

When transistor technology was invented in the 1960s and 1970s, it paved the way for much simpler, user-friendly electrolysis equipment that is now in use and still evolving. Since the dawn of epilator technology many issues have moved to the forefront of an electrologist's training such as physiological reasons for hirsutism, hair and skin issues, biology, bacteriology, and sterilization. For example, following the lead of other health-care professions in the early 1980s in response to blood-borne viruses such as HIV, many electrologists began to use presterilized, disposable needles.

Figure 7. Uniprobe Electolysis Probe

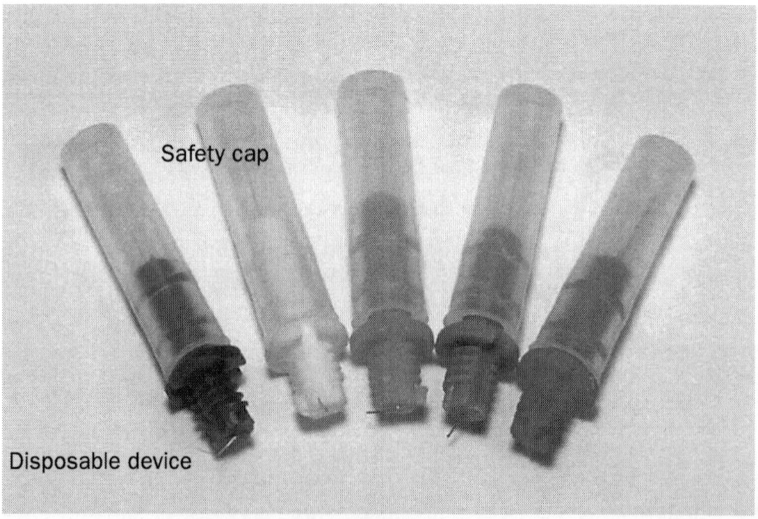

This combined probe and cap makes a sanitary disposable unit. It is color-coded for different needle sizes. Photo Credit: www.uniprobe.com, inventor of the patented device.

||||||||||||||||||||||||||||||||||||||||||||||||||||||||||||||||||||||||||
Treating Ingrown Hairs and Folliculitis
Electrolysis treatments can actually eliminate ingrown hairs and folliculitis. For some electrologists, treating these kinds of problems really is just business as usual. If you are experiencing problems with ingrown hairs or folliculitis, look into the training and skill level of your electrologist. A trained professional can help, since removing the hair improves whatever has been aggravating the skin.
||||||||||||||||||||||||||||||||||||||||||||||||||||||||||||||||||||||||||

THE PAIN MYTH

Electrolysis is considered less painful than waxing, a lot less painful than tweezer like devices, and a lot more comfortable from a patient's perspective than either a Pap smear or getting your teeth cleaned. It is not painless though, and comparisons can hopefully give you a sense of the pain or discomfort threshold levels.

For destruction to take place within the hair follicle, some sensation has to be involved; however, the electrologist can make adjustments in the timing and/or intensity of the current and can find a setting comfortable for you. Topical analgesics are available over-the-counter and by prescription for those who are worried about any discomfort, but in most cases, electrologists find that their patients simply don't need them. With proper technique, settings, and up-to-date equipment, you may feel very little discomfort aside from a slight heat sensation at the bottom of the follicle. Many first-time patients say, "If I'd have known it was like this, I'd have done it years ago."

The higher the electrical current used, the greater the discomfort. Sometimes electrologists will use a high current on a particularly stubborn hair, but even so, the pain factor is not great. Generally speaking, the higher the intensity of the current, the greater the destruction of the follicle. It is an electrologist's responsibility to find the appropriate degree of intensity: one strong enough to destroy the follicle without harming the skin or causing too much discomfort. Communicate your discomfort level clearly so that your electrologist can remedy the problem or use an analgesic.

An electrologist should also have good manual dexterity: no shaking or arthritic movement. He or she should also have excellent unaided vision or use equipment with magnification. Go ahead and ask; it is your body. You also should not feel obliged to continue with a technician if you do not wish to.

SAFETY CONCERNS

Many women assume that because electrolysis involves an electrical current that it is unsafe or even carcinogenic (cancer-causing). Studies have repeatedly shown that electrolysis does not put you at risk for cancer and no studies to date have shown that electrolysis is unsafe. Using electricity in electrolysis is not the same thing as radiation, although these two are sometimes confused.

Nor does electrolysis affect a nonpregnant woman's capacity to breastfeed. This means that hair removal around the nipple area is considered absolutely safe for those of you who are not pregnant. If you are pregnant, so long as you avoid electrolysis treatment on the abdomen or breasts during the last trimester, it is considered safe. This is not to say that pregnant women have experienced negative side effects, but restricting third trimester treatment is done as a precaution. Some electrologists may ask you to seek your physician's approval as a further precaution.

On the other end, technicians need to be scrupulous with their craft and with you. After your treatment, if you notice any swelling beyond what is explained to you, or any discoloration, seek immediate care from a physician to prevent scarring and to minimize injury.

AFTERCARE

It is natural to experience a bit of redness or swelling after an electrolysis treatment, and your electrologist has an obligation to inform you of proper aftercare procedures to aid the skin in healing. In cases of extremely sensitive skin, the best aftercare is no care, to simply leave the skin alone. In most cases, after treatment, an electrologist applies an antiseptic that is specifically prepared for electrolysis. The antiseptic often contains one or a combination of the following: tea tree oil, camphor, or 3 percent hydrogen peroxide. Then, a healing agent is commonly applied, such as aloe vera gel, vitamin C serum, or an antibacterial ointment, or cream.

Ask your electrologist to provide you with oral or written instructions about aftercare procedures that are specific to you. Use caution with these procedures at home and check with a qualified professional if you have any doubts. For most women this aftercare treatment is sufficient, but if you are having problems with healing, consult a dermatologist for the best postcare or pretreatment approach and share these suggestions with your electrologist. If healing is a concern, ask the electrologist you interview (see the section on consultation) about his or her experience working with your skin type.

TIMING IS EVERYTHING

Electrolysis requires a time commitment. Do not rush it or be impatient. If you decide to go for it, you have to be sure that you rule out any underlying hormonal problem, otherwise you may wind up forever "chasing hairs." Although electrolysis can destroy existing hairs, it can't control the new hairs being stimulated to grow or that become terminal hairs.

The common misconception about electrolysis is that you need only one treatment per hair. Once is not enough. This is because hair can take from several weeks to several months to fully cycle through (i.e., complete the three-stage growth cycle). Repeated treatments may be necessary to catch the hair in the active growth stage—the anagen phase.

By catching the hairs in a growing phase, it is easier to kill the follicle. In fact, when you are undergoing electrolysis treatment, you might be instructed to return as soon as you see the hair return. This is largely because electrologists realize that some of us cannot deal with the returning hairs and may be tempted to pull them out before treatment. In that case, you would have to wait for the hair to cycle through again. Hair follicles can take several weeks to several months (depending on body area) to transition. Someone who has treatments two or three times a year won't make the same kind of progress as someone who is treated more frequently.

Waiting a lengthy amount of time between treatments will result in a longer killing process because the hair may go into its resting phase. For more details about hair growth cycles, see chapter 2. An electrolysis treatment can undoubtedly coincide with the hair cell's other two stages, although the anagen phase is the easiest for destruction to take place. A competent electrologist can still get at the nourishment source at the bottom of the follicle in the other two stages; nevertheless, you have to keep returning for treatments until the hair's targeted growth cells are destroyed and won't grow back. In addition, if you have inadvertently strengthened your hair follicles from years of tweezing, waxing, yanking, and so on, you will likely need more treatments to achieve permanence.

If you are working on an area where you have a low tolerance for hair, once treatment begins you may need two or three treatments a week for two months before the growth subsides. Be careful not to overtreat the skin by repeatedly treating a small area that makes you feel self-conscious.

As treatments progress, the hair takes longer and longer to come back and appears finer and finer until they are unable to reproduce. The time span between appointments eventually lengthens, until you'll find that you only need to go once every six to eight weeks for just a few finer strands of hair. Women with moderate hair growth are looking at an average time commitment of nine months to a year before hair in a certain area ceases to grow altogether or ceases to be a major problem. The visits every six to eight weeks "clean up" a few fine strands that have yet to be fully zapped.

Your time commitment depends on so many factors, such as how much hair is present, how quickly your hair grows, how often you go for treatment, skin sensitivity, hormonal changes, method used, and so on. The electrologist's skill also has a bearing on how quickly the hairs grow or do not grow back. An experienced electrologist knows how to successfully reach the hair growth cells in the different phases and to skillfully deliver the correct current.

COST AND CONVENIENCE

Electrolysis is not cheap, but it is not cost prohibitive. It is charged by units of time and the cost of treatment varies quite a bit in the United States. Fifteen minutes is usually about $15 to $25, depending on where you live. Sometimes an electrologist charges a dollar a minute, which can be more cost effective, but most do not work this way.

For example, an electrologist may not want to treat the upper lip area for more than fifteen minutes at a time, no matter how much hair is present. The upper lip is very sensitive and the skin is easily aggravated. Hair follicles are also very close together and it is important not to treat too many contiguous hairs in this area. Therefore, expecting that one treatment clears an upper lip is not realistic. Keep in mind that electrolysis requires time and, above all, patience.

If you cannot tolerate having any hair remaining, or any new hair appearing, you may need to schedule fifteen minutes two to three times a week when you first begin treatment. This can add up. If you have a lot of hair, you may initially require longer treatments to the hair under control.

Generally speaking, the first fifteen minutes are the most costly (due to fixed expenses such as needles, antiseptic products, aftercare preparations, and so on). Additional time can usually be scheduled at a slightly lower rate. There are offices where this is not the case, so do your homework.

If necessary, a thirty- or forty-five-minute appointment once a week can prove to be more time efficient as well as more cost effective than a short visit. If you are on a budget, it is best to concentrate on a small area first, and then move on to other areas as your budget and time permit. By aggressively treating your one area, you save money in the long term.

For whatever reasons, if you can only budget a fifteen-minute treatment every two to three weeks (and you really should be going in for forty-five minutes each week) and seriously want to remove your hair, should you still start treatment? Absolutely. The process takes longer, but you can still make progress. It can't be stressed enough: Electrolysis takes time and patience.

Given the permanence of electrolysis, it is affordable for most middle- and upper-income women. Unfortunately, this procedure is still costly for lower-income women and, therefore, is often not an option. Less frequent sessions, however, can still destroy the regenerative ability of the follicle, although it may take longer to fully disable the follicle and thus achieve permanence.

Depending on the extent of your hair growth and the kindness of your electrologist, you may be able to negotiate a lower fee, but professionals usually can't afford this because they have business overhead and mouths to feed, too. Most women do the math and come up with a compromise. Remove the most unsightly and problematic hairs with electrolysis, and opt for another method for larger areas. The most popular area for electrolysis is the face: chin, sideburns, and upper lip.

Also, keep in mind that tweezing hairs you are already treating with electrolysis is like throwing money down the drain because you are strengthening the roots and making the hair more difficult for the electrologist to destroy, no matter how skilled he or she is.

SETTING UP A CONSULTATION

Before visiting an electrologist, it is important to rule out an underlying hormonal cause for hair growth. Once you have addressed the possibility of underlying causes for hirsutism or have begun to deal with them, the next step is researching electrologists. It is important to find a credentialed electrologist with whom you feel comfortable. Prior to treatment, be sure to have a consultation with as many technicians as possible to choose the best one for you. Do not rush.

Unwanted Hair and Hirsutism

Finding a Qualified Provider

Where do you find an electrologist? If a medical doctor is treating you for hirsutism, ask him or her for a referral. The American Electrology Association (www.aea.org) and the Society for Clinical & Medical Hair Removal (www.scmhr.org) have state-by-state directories. Also ask friends, family, and neighbors for recommendations. Many city and regional papers give awards based on reader voting, so that is another way to begin searching. Do your research carefully. A coupon might sound good at first, but it is worthless if the technician is not right for you.

What to Ask a Potential Electrologist

During the consultation, you'll need to make your goals clear. Ask yourself these questions ahead of time:

1. What areas do you want to treat?
2. What are your expectations for your time commitment?
3. What results do you expect?

A frank discussion at the outset will save you aggravation. Consider asking your candidates the following questions:

What, realistically, do you expect in terms of time and results?
This is an important area to be in alignment. If your expectations are different from what the electrologist assesses to be the reality, you may be disappointed.

How do I manage the hair growth area between appointments?
Your best bet is to shave, trim, or cut the hairs between appointments. You should be instructed to resist plucking, tweezing, waxing, threading, or any other epilation on treated hairs that grow back. This will waste your money and time, as it will only strengthen the roots and impede much of the progress you've made thus far.

How long should I wait between appointments?
The longer you wait, the harder it will be to achieve optimum results. Treating the hair while it is in the active growing phase is important, and will speed up the process of destruction. Regularity of treatments is also important, so try

to devise an appointment schedule based on what sort of regrowth you feel you can tolerate and what results you'd like to see in the long term. On the other end of the spectrum, avoid overtreating the area.

What are your qualifications and training?
You want an experienced electrologist who has had adequate and proper training. See the next section on credentials and licensing.

How did you become interested in this profession?
It is always good to know whether an electrologist's interest in the profession stemmed from his or her own battle with hirsutism. This often allows for more comfort between you and your electrologist—who you may be seeing a lot more than even your doctor.

Have you dealt with my particular problem areas before and how frequently with clients with my skin tone?
Because certain skin tones or areas require different treatment approaches (olive-toned skin, for example, is prone to pigment changes and may require more diligent aftercare), it is recommended that you find an electrologist who has worked with clients with hair and skin like yours.

What should I expect in terms of discomfort or pain?
Look for the electrologist to describe something similar to what has been discussed earlier in this chapter, for instance, "There is discomfort. It should not be particularly painful and if you are experiencing pain be sure to tell me immediately."

Do you use sterile, disposable needles and sterile forceps?
Forceps are tweezers that remove the hair once it is been treated. Electrologists who do not use disposable needles or sterile forceps are not adhering to infection control standards for the electrology profession, regardless of whether or not your state permits it. It is even better if they show you the packages. A needle soaking in a solution is not one that the technician disposes after every use, as is the standard.

CREDENTIALS AND LICENSING ARE EVERYTHING

Those states in the United States that require licensing also require electrologists to display their license. If you have to look for the license, it is a bad sign. Electrology is licensed in most of the United States, but not in all states and not in Canada. Right now, if you live in a state or a Canadian region that does not require licensing, ask if your electrologist has the Certified Professional Electrologist (CPE) credential.

It is also not enough that the spa or treatment center is licensed to practice business in your state; individual technicians must be credentialed. Electrologists with training and international certification proudly present their credentials, the same as dentists display diplomas on the wall. Electrologists of any merit are certified, and if they are not, you risk scarring or damaging your skin. If a practitioner is an apprentice, he or she may be practicing on you and you need to know that ahead of time. In this case, the fees should be lower and the apprentice should be supervised while administering the treatment.

Credentialed electrologists have a CPE certification from the American Electrology Association (AEA), or a Certified Clinical Electrologist (CCE) or a Certified Medical Electrologist (CME) from the Society for Clinical & Medical Hair Removal, Inc. CCE is the entry-level certification and CME is the next level.

Canadian electrologists may appear to be similarly certified because the CPE is in fact an international credential of the American Electrology Association (AEA); however, the Canadian CPE is not a part of the AEA's international board certification program. It is a peer certification of the Federation of Canadian Electrolysis Associations (FCEA), not an international board certification. So if you live in Canada and you are using certification as a means of evaluating your practitioner, ask careful questions about his or her training and safety standards before you opt for treatment.

In the United States, the CPE exams are developed, written, administered, and proctored by Chauncey Group International, a subsidiary of the Educational Testing Service (ETS), the administrators of the SAT exams and other board-certification exams. The CPE credential indicates that your electrologist has voluntarily met an established norm and is committed to continuing education to maintain board-certified status. Electrologists from as far as Australia, Croatia, Germany, Israel, Japan, Luxembourg, Puerto Rico, and the United Kingdom, among others, have come to the United States to take the CPE exam. The International Commission for Hair Removal Certification provides the competency-based certification examinations for the CCE and the CME.

While you are checking credentials, also ask if the electrologist adheres to the AEA's Infection Control Standards for the Practice of Electrology. An electrologist—regardless of where he or she practices—is considered a health-care practitioner. This means that whether this individual is trained in what is considered a conventional or an unconventional manner, charging a fee for services implies there are standards of what is legally referred to as "awareness and proficiency," which clients have a right to expect. Thus, any kind of health-care professional who earns a salary has legal and ethical duties to stay educated, informed, and up to date on all aspects of his or her profession.

CHAPTER 11

LASER HAIR REMOVAL: WHAT YOU NEED TO KNOW

Laser treatment is sometimes presented as an alternative to electrolysis; however, it does not have the same effect. Laser treatment does remove hair, and if you have large areas of hair you want to remove, you may want to seriously consider it because it treats large areas of hair at once, not one follicle at a time as does electrolysis. As long as your expectations are realistic, it may work for you.

Laser hair removal results in permanent hair reduction rather than permanent hair removal. The laser method is an effective way to remove hair temporarily for three months to a year, and even longer for some hair. It is most effective on people with fair skin and dark hair; however, new devices are constantly in development for other types of skin and hair. In some instances, the hair does grow back a little finer, and in some cases, the follicle is damaged so that growth is slow, but it is important to realize that generally the hair does grow back.

HOW LASER HAIR REMOVAL WORKS

A laser device is placed against your skin and irradiates it with an intense, pulsating beam of hot light. The beam targets the melanin, the dark pigment contained within the hair shaft. When the beam hits your hair follicle, it destroys the shaft, essentially cooking it. This process causes inflammation in the hair follicle and the reaction sends your hair into the resting (telogen) phase. Your hair growth cells are not dead; they are instead resting. The irradiated hairs grow back slower and often the follicle is altered so that it now produces lighter, shorter, finer (vellus) hairs.

Laser treatment only works on hair that is in the active stage (anagen), so hair in the other transitional and resting stages (catagen and telogen) continue to cycle through normally and grow out and through your skin, necessitating multiple treatments to catch hair in the active stage. And because the hair growth cells are still alive, they grow back within a year, generally in about four months. Studies of laser treatment show a 50 percent growth decrease in the hair follicles of the treated area due to scarring of the follicles.

However, a single treatment may produce complete hair regrowth within two to six months.

The key to using laser hair removal is the contrast in color between your skin and hair. When the treatment doesn't work, it is because the pigment in your skin absorbs the laser, instead of the pigment in your hair. Most of the laser energy is said to pass right through light-colored skin without doing any harm. But if you have dark skin, it is more difficult for the laser operator to avoid injuring the melanin pigment in the surface of your skin. The beam must be administered only long enough to heat the hair follicle and not so it heats the surrounding skin, which can change the pigmentation or burn you.

Grouped into the category of laser hair removal and used by some practitioners is a nonlaser, pulsed light source. It is used for other purposes besides hair removal as the light wavelengths are broad and target more than pigment. The device is often called an intense pulse light (IPL). It can be dangerous because it requires a lot of power to work. Studies have shown that the thermal lasers are more effective than using only the light source.

Today, three main types of lasers are used depending on your hair's thickness and your skin color. Differences among laser devices include their cooling mechanisms. The technology changes fairly quickly so you want to learn about the best devices for you during consultations with various practitioners who use different devices.

IS LASER HAIR REMOVAL RIGHT FOR YOU?

From the *Consumer Guide to Laser Hair Removal*:

> Lasers are not for everyone, and their proper use requires great expertise. Consumers contemplating laser hair removal require education to properly evaluate if and where to have laser hair removal performed. Many competing technologies exist. Several are already outmoded, and others offer particular advantages for certain patient populations.
>
> The absolute requirement is that one's hair must be darker than the surrounding skin. Additionally, very darkly pigmented people absorb too much laser energy in their skin and are not ideal candidates. Tanned patients with light hair are not candidates. Tanned patients with dark hair should wait until their tan fades before they are treated. Lastly the treatment cost should be within reach of the patient.

Unwanted Hair and Hirsutism

This guide is sponsored by the Institute of Laser Medicine and can be found at www.consumerlaserguide.com. It is difficult to find sufficient understandable information about laser treatment on the Internet. Many Web sites have commercial interests and are trying to gain your business, even those sponsored by medical centers and doctors. There is a lot of money to be made in laser hair treatment. This book can help to fill a void of objective information.

The trouble with laser treatment is that it is sold as "permanent" when it is not, which has consumers doling out thousands of dollars for a method that is not permanent. Legitimate laser practitioners will tell you that the technique is not permanent and does not make guarantees. However, even the most genuine sources promote general information in the best-case scenario, which may not have the best outcome for your specific hair and skin type.

Laser devices have been FDA approved with language that is misleading: "permanent" hair reduction. But it is just that—a reduction. Many people are satisfied with the slow regrowth or that some hairs grow back finer or lighter, so it is not an issue that the hair is not permanently removed. Nevertheless, it is important to know that laser hair removal is not permanent and that it requires frequent treatment for slow regrowth and regular maintenance to remove the new hairs as they grow back.

The FDA defines *reduction* as "30 percent or more after a treatment regimen for a period of time longer than the regrowth cycle." In other words, only 30 percent of your treated hair needs to have a reduction in growth, and only for four to twelve months, depending on the area of your body. That leaves up to 70 percent growing back right away, or according to your genetic makeup. For more specific information, visit the FDA Web site at www.fda.gov/cdrh/consumer/laserfacts.html.

You may be surprised to read this statistic because laser therapy is prominently advertised and frequently endorsed by doctors. Physicians are usually mandated by state law to supervise this procedure, which is often performed in their office—that's why you see doctors' advertising that they perform laser treatment.

It seems that even some researchers and physicians not involved with hair removal are misled by the word "permanence." There are many instances in contemporary medical literature where physicians recommend laser therapy as treatment for hair removal, and not just as temporary management.

Likewise, much of the medical literature says that electrolysis is painful when comparing it to laser hair removal, while failing to compare it to other painful methods such as waxing. The danger for patients is that doctors read medical studies and use the information to diagnose and treat their patients, so you can easily receive misleading information about laser treatment.

There is also a lack of medical information about the side effects of laser hair removal available for both the general public and health-care providers. Particularly lacking is the fact that laser hair removal only works on certain demographics of people. Some in the hair removal field believe that because many physicians are required to supervise laser hair removal and that many perform it themselves, they know more about it than about other hair removal methods and therefore recommend laser treatment less objectively than they do others. Be advised that your doctor may not have a full range of information and be prepared to make your own decisions about hair removal.

Is Enough Ever Enough?

There are no research findings indicating when a client has received enough laser treatment to slow hair growth, and it differs from person to person depending on their hair. You may want follow-up treatment every six months or so as the hair grows back in. Generally speaking, according to the Mayo Foundation for Medical Education and Research, for one area of your body you can "expect to undergo six to eight treatments spaced six to eight weeks apart to achieve good reduction of hair and slowing of hair regrowth. Then, you will likely undergo periodic maintenance treatments." If you are of Mediterranean descent, chances are you are looking at more time and money.

If you see an advertisement that appears to be too good to be true, it probably is. A laser treatment facility cannot guarantee the rate of your hair regrowth, and if a physician or other technician tries to do so, he or she is using a crystal ball and you should steer clear.

A BRIEF HISTORY OF LASER HAIR REMOVAL

The laser hype started in 1995 when the company ThermoLase licensed its hair removal laser (a SoftLight NG:YAG) to physicians and spas throughout the United States. This system emitted a red light that was absorbed by a black carbon lotion applied topically to freshly waxed skin. It was marketed as permanent and painless; it was neither. To avoid pain, a topical anesthetic was applied prior to treatment, which means treatment was not painless.

After treatment, a "sunburn" type of pain resulted in some cases. As for the permanence claim, a clinical study revealed that SoftLight was "100 percent temporary" and that hair regrowth in all treated areas occurred by the sixth month.

On May 26, 1998, a class action complaint was filed by client Laurel Tester against ThermoLase in California. Tester was angry that the laser product was advertised as long lasting, when in fact it was not. ThermoLase quietly settled out of court in late 1998. All studies done on laser techniques to date show the same results: pricey without the permanence.

Ruby laser systems became popular after the SoftLight, and worked the same way but did not require pretreatment with any sort of topical application. We are now seeing what are called the fourth generation of laser products, which are diode systems, emitting a red light that is absorbed by the melanin in the follicle.

The technology is developing all the time so it is worthwhile to see what new treatment is available, just as it is important that whoever you hire is using the latest and best technology—approved by the FDA—for your skin type.

PREPARATION
For Women with Dark Skin
Your skin will absorbs the laser energy—which is heat—since it has a lot of pigment, exposing you to discoloration, blistering, and burning. The technology has improved so that a competent technician can remove the hair much better than in the past. The recommended laser is ND:YAG. However, if you are dark-skinned and have fine, light hair, laser treatment is not effective. If you are dark-skinned and seek out laser hair removal, be sure to find a center or technician that specializes in your skin type. One potentially positive feature is that dark-skinned people often have coarse hair, and coarse hair is easier to remove.

For Women with Blond or Red Hair
Because the laser works through your hair's pigment, if the hair you seek to remove is blond, white, or red, it does not work.

Tanning

Do not schedule your laser hair removal session after a trip to the beach. Laser treatment is not compatible with tanning, especially if your skin becomes darker than your hair. Wait for your tan to fade completely, then the laser will be more effective. In addition, a tan increases the risk of the laser causing blisters and discoloring your skin. Generally, avoid exposing the treatment area to the sun for four to six weeks before your scheduled treatment. The same rule applies for spray tans.

Preparing the Area

Do not wax, thread, tweeze, or otherwise yank your hair for three weeks before treatment. Do not bleach your hair because it needs to be darker than your skin color. Also, do not use electrolysis in this area for three weeks prior to laser treatment. Shaving, cutting, and trimming are okay.

Diet

Yes, it is true. Your diet does influence laser treatment. Eating carrots, orange or yellow squash, vitamins with vitamin A—any substance with beta carotene (vitamin A)—produces a subtle orange or yellow color in your skin. This pigment in your skin absorbs the laser; therefore, more of the laser energy goes into the skin and less into the hair follicle, thereby making it less effective. For more effective treatment, do not eat orange or yellow food or take supplements with vitamin A for several months.

Pain

Laser therapy is considered less painful than electrolysis, but it is still painful. There is intense heat being applied to your body. As with any hair removal procedure, the range varies with the body part and person.

SAFETY CONCERNS

As with any hair removal procedure, there are risks and side effects. The following are some of the risks involved with laser hair removal:

- *Radiation risks.* There is no risk of cancer. The lasers approved by the FDA for use in hair removal use nonionizing radiation, similar to radiation from lightbulbs, radio waves, and fire flames. It is not the same radiation used by X-rays, for instance. Nevertheless, be alert to any undiagnosed skin lesions because laser hair removal may remove a lesion that is important for diagnosis. If you have a mole or other skin growth that has caused you or a doctor concern, follow up with its diagnosis before removing it by laser treatment.
- *Skin discoloration.* Your skin can become dark after treatment, which is called hyperpigmentation. Although usually temporary, it can be long lasting or permanent in some instances. In contrast, if you are dark skinned, lightening can occur, which is called *hypopigmentation.*
- *Other toxins.* The smoky plume emitted by the laser hair removal method contains toxic gases and vapors, which can cause upper respiratory tract problems for staff. Also, viruses such as HPV, HIV, herpes, and TB can be transmitted via the plume (which forms as a result of vaporizing the hair shaft) from the patient to the operator if the vacuum suction is not properly working, so notify the operator if you have a transmittable virus.
- *Skin burning.* The type of laser must be matched to your skin type; otherwise, you can be burned as the laser finds the pigment in your skin and causes thermal damage (heat). Asian people often have latent pigmentation, which is not obvious to the eye, and they should be careful. The levels of pigment in olive-skinned people make them more difficult, too. Good technicians will do a test spot first and wait for a few days, but no longer than a week, to see the effects.
- *Acne.* Research has found that this side effect occurs in 6 percent of patients and is more likely with the ND:YAG laser than the others (14 percent). It is more common in younger patients. There is no correlation between acne with the topical cooling gels or gender of the client; it affects everyone the same.

AFTERCARE

It is natural to experience redness or swelling after a laser treatment. Your provider has an obligation to inform you of proper aftercare procedures to aid your skin in healing. Immediately after the treatment the technician or doctor should apply a cooling agent, such as an ointment or gel, and a cold compress or ice. Gel from an aloe plant or pure aloe gel without chemicals is recommended as something you can apply yourself at home. In the long term, gel from a plant is more cost effective and environmentally friendly than gel from a bottle.

You should avoid direct exposure to sunlight for a period of time after treatment, from a few days to a few weeks, depending on the laser device. This is not the kind of procedure to try right before a planned beach vacation.

Follow your practitioner's instructions about what hair removal techniques to use between treatments, as they can affect your next treatment. Ask for oral or written instructions about specific aftercare procedures for you. For most women, the recommended aftercare treatment is sufficient, but if you have problems with healing, consult a dermatologist for the best pretreatment and aftercare approaches and share these suggestions with your laser technician or doctor.

COST AND CONVENIENCE

Laser hair removal can be cost prohibitive for many women. An area such as the bikini area starts at about $450, wheareas a larger area, such as the legs, can cost up to $1,000. This is just for the first treatment. Many clinics offer a "cost per body area" deal, meaning that you pay one fee for several treatments. There is no guarantee that you will be "done" after the deal expires, so keep this in mind as well as the fact it is not permanent, so you may be back in two years.

Look out for hidden costs. Sometimes a treatment fee is just for the doctor's labor, but there are also costs for add-ons. Be sure you know all the costs ahead of time and plan on at least four sessions. Also, the clinic must be upfront about whether the fee is for the doctor or whomever the doctor is supervising. If you are going to pay all that money at a doctor's office, you may want a real doctor; alternatively, you may get a great deal by hiring a certified technician who charges less.

Costs differ from one region of the country to the next, just as they do for health care in general. There may even be differences between one suburb and the next, versus a city with more competition or a high-priced city. And do not assume a high-priced spa is better quality. Always try to negotiate a package price for a lower rate, or a discount on maintenance treatments, wherever you go.

SETTING UP A CONSULTATION

Make an appointment for a consultation with a few places. During the consultation, cover the following:

1. Ask for the technician or doctor's credentials. If the clinic promotes a doctor's care, be sure to ask who exactly is performing the hair removal procedure and meet that person. Sometimes nurses or nurse practitioners will perform the removal but you have to pay a doctor's prices. Ask the actual practitioner for his or her credentials.
2. If your state or province requires licensing, make sure the practitioner's license is displayed prominently. If it is not, leave.
3. Ask how long the practitioner has been practicing and what are his or her qualifications, including training.
4. Ask how long the practitioner has had experience with your hair or skin type.
5. Be sure they discuss aftercare with you.
6. Ask what kind of lasers or devices they use. Be sure they have the kind most effective for your hair and skin.
7. See if you feel comfortable with the practitioner.
8. If the practitioner mentions or promotes guarantees for permanent hair removal they are not legitimate and you should keep looking.
9. The practitioner should recommend performing a spot test and suggest you come back within a week to see the results. If he or she doesn't, mark this person off the list. You don't need to get a spot test right then and there, but you should have one before the treatments are scheduled.

CREDENTIALS AND REGULATIONS ARE EVERYTHING

The laser can easily damage your tissues. You must have someone qualified to use the device and, for the best results, you must have the appropriate laser.

Unfortunately, many states do not have regulations governing the use of lasers for hair removal. This can expose you to horrible scarring or other skin damage by unqualified technicians. In states with no regulations, laser removal is popping up on every corner in salons and spas that are competing with each other through aggressive advertising. Warning: Technicians who are trained at a sales seminar are not trained appropriately, and they are probably not certified, either. Only a few states currently require anyone performing laser hair removal to be certified, even doctors.

On the other hand, most states that have laser hair removal regulations require a physician's supervision or some kind of relationship with a physician. However, this does not mean the physician is specially trained to use the devices or is certified. Only a few states currently require anyone performing laser hair removal to be certified.

There are turf wars going on over performing laser hair removal. You can tell by the prices that there is money to be made in this business, and as hairlessness becomes more and more fashionable, people want to cash in. If you look on the Internet, you can find many Web sites with doctors telling you to go to a doctor and not to a technician, even though sometimes laypeople have better training and credentials and more experience. Dermatologists and plastic surgeons, in particular, offer laser hair removal. However, there are other highly trained specialists who can provide the procedure, and they are usually less expensive than physicians.

The credentials of people practicing laser technology have been all over the map. In the United States, there are no federal regulations about who may or may not use a laser for hair removal. According to the FDA, "surgical devices" (a category that encompasses laser hair removal technology) are considered prescription devices by default. Nevertheless, they may be used by any type of practicing doctor as state law allows (or restricts), and many states have no rules. For more information, please see FDA 21 CFR (Code of Federal Regulations) Section 801.109. Some states are beginning to regulate and require certification, but most do not. See chapter 11 for more information about business regulation and consumer protection.

Finding a Qualified Provider

You do not have to guess who is qualified to use a laser device on your body. An international nonprofit trade association, the Society for Clinical & Medical Hair Removal, Inc., certifies people properly trained in laser hair removal all over the world, including safety, the physics of laser use on skin and hair, types of laser, and aftercare. The credential is called CLHRP—Certified Laser Hair Removal Professional. The International Commission for Hair Removal Certification provides the competency-based certification examinations. A few states require this certification, but otherwise it is voluntary, so if you don't see the certificate displayed, ask the technician or doctor if she or he has one. The Society for Clinical & Medical Hair Removal has a directory of certified technicians and doctors in the United States, Canada, Lebanon, and Japan. Their Web site is www.scmrh.org.

Ask how long the provider has been in practice, or how long the salon has been performing laser hair removal, and check the provider's record if possible with your state government or the Better Business Bureau.

CHAPTER 12

PROTECTING YOURSELF FROM SKIN DAMAGE: RISKS AND REGULATIONS

Unfortunately, for people in the United States, there are no uniform regulations or consumer protections for hair removal, perhaps because it is something that affects primarily women. Experts believe that much of the damage done by in-home devices is not tracked by government agencies, thereby making it more difficult for you to make effective decisions. And more and more devices appear on the market, claiming everything from laser technology to laserlike heat and electrolysis.

If you have questions regarding claims about a specific device, call the FDA's Office of Consumer Affairs at 1-800-532-4440. Also, it is important to note that the term "clearance to market" promoted on some products is not the same as receiving FDA approval. Some product manufacturers advertise FDA approval when what they have actually been approved for clearance to market. For information on how to distinguish between the two categories, call the FDA 800 number or visit www.fda.gov/cdrh/consumer/laserfacts.html.

SPAS, SALONS, AND MEDICAL CENTERS

As described in chapter 7, it is easy to find a business that will remove your hair. They are everywhere. However, just because the business has a fancy name, does not mean the people removing your hair are trained properly. Take extra caution if you use a business in a state with few or no regulations, as there are not many repercussions if its employees burn or hurt you. Do not be embarrassed to ask for credentials.

You can be seriously hurt by an unqualified electrologist or laser technician. An improperly trained electrologist can cause a keloid (permanent skin scar) if the needle is left in the follicle too long. He or she can also cause intense pain. Laser treatment can burn your skin. Untrained waxers can cause intense pain, temporary infection or inflammation, and skin discoloration—not to mention giving you a shape you don't want. If your skin appears swollen or discolored, seek medical attention immediately. This advice also applies to hair removal techniques you try at home.

One rule of thumb is to find a salon that has been in business for many years and has customers. Businesses that have been sued are likely go out of business.

LASER TREATMENTS

Laser treatments are used for everything from cataracts to removing wine stains. Here is a statement from the FDA:

> The popularity of laser hair removal has increasingly grown, prompting many laser manufacturers to conduct research and seek FDA clearance for their lasers for this indication. The market is growing so quickly that the FDA cannot maintain an up-to-date list of all laser manufacturers whose devices have been cleared for hair removal, as this list continues to change. To learn if a specific manufacturer has received FDA clearance, you can check FDA's Web site at http://www.fda.gov/cdrh/databases.html under the 510(k) database. You will need to know the manufacturer or device name of the laser. You can also call FDA's Center for Devices and Radiological Health, Consumer Staff, at 240-276-3103; fax your request to 240-276-3151; or send an e-mail to: DSMICA@cdrh.fda.gov.
>
> Manufacturers should be aware that receiving an FDA clearance for general permission to market their devices does not permit them to advertise the lasers for either hair removal or wrinkle treatment, even though hair removal or wrinkle treatment may be a by-product of any cleared laser procedure. Further, manufacturers may not claim that laser hair removal is either painless or permanent unless the FDA determines that there are sufficient data to demonstrate such results.

Is Laser Treatment Experimental Therapy?

Laser hair removal has only been around only since the mid-1990s, and therefore is relatively new and considered by many experts to be experimental therapy. As more and more devices are developed and marketed, there is a natural gap between their beginnings and their long-term proven safety and effectiveness. Experimental medical therapy on female subjects has a long history of abusing women, who again may find themselves harmed given that mostly women seek laser hair removal and it is considered experimental.

Susan Sherwin, a professor of medical ethics and author of *No Longer Patient: Feminist Ethics & Health Care* (1992), writes: "In case after case we find that women receive treatments that have been falsely represented as safe . . . with no warnings or explanations" (p. 168). According to Sherwin, "Women's relatively powerless positions in society make it a matter of particular importance that we guard against the likelihood that their health is sacrificed to the financial interests of the [manufacturer]" (p. 169).

To make matters worse, innovation drives product development; therefore you may unwittingly be a subject to a new, innovative technique. The device may be approved for use, but the way it is used on you and others may be experimental. Be aware: It is better to stick to established treatment methods used on standard parts of your body.

Unfortunately, people anxious to receive a promising new treatment may find themselves human subjects of medical research. Informed consent is one way to guard against possible harms associated with experimental therapies. Informed consent means that when you are being given a treatment—be it experimental or standard—your health-care practitioner (in this case, the person performing the laser treatment) ought to disclose, first and foremost, whether the treatment is experimental or standard.

DISCLOSURE STATEMENTS

Most state laws require clients to sign a consent form for any kind of health care. This does not mean states that do not consider electrolysis as a type of health care require the client's written consent; however, it is a good practice for a reputable technician to follow. You have probably seen these consent forms at the doctor's or dentist's office. Please read these forms very carefully. For informed consent to take place, there must be full disclosure of what treatment entails, you must understand the information being disclosed, and your treatment must be voluntary—no coercion involved.

Ask about anything you do not understand. It is your right, and good practitioners do not mind explaining the procedures to you. If the doctor or technician acts as if you do not need to know or should not care, walk away.

CHAPTER 13

IMPROVING YOUR BODY IMAGE —HAIR AND ALL

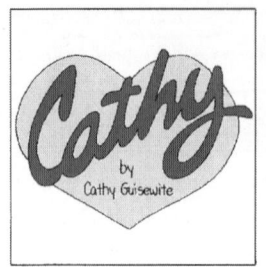

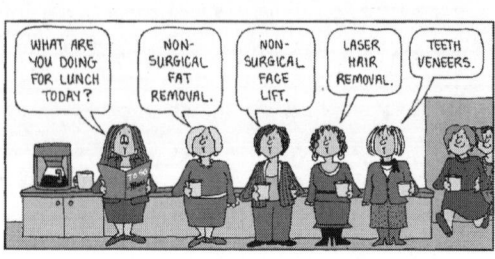

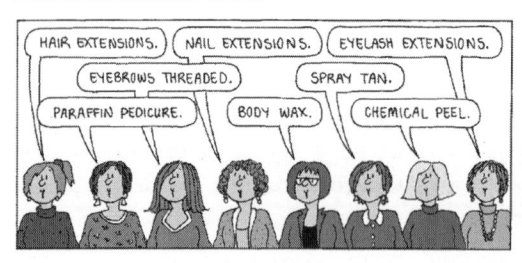

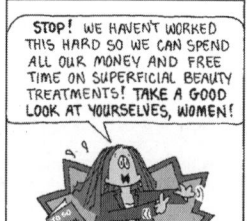

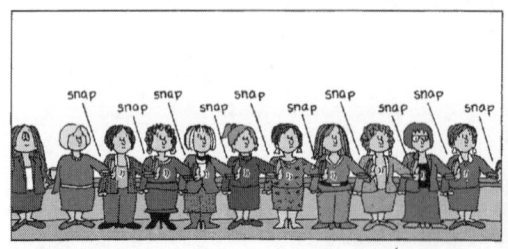

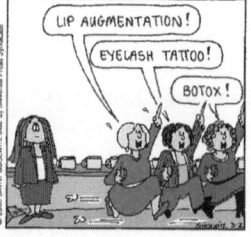

Cathy © 2008 Cathy Guisewite. Reprinted by permission of Universal Press Syndicate. All rights reserved.

The vast majority of women seldom stop thinking about their body. Most of us have an unhealthy fixation on our weight and general physical appearance. For those of us struggling with unwanted hair, it can aggravate negative perceptions we already have about our body.

Every day women wake up to a powerful psychological attack on our appearance. In the same way that commercial media plays into distorted body sizes by making women of appropriate weight feel "fat," thus contributing to a rise in eating disorders, society also plays a role in making women with appropriate amounts of body hair feel "abnormal."

How do we measure up? We can't help but reflect these images on ourselves. They are thrown at us at every turn through billboards, television, magazines, Internet news, Web sites, and newspapers. There is no escaping the sexualized images that are created to titillate men into buying, reading, or using some product. Unfortunately, the images are peddled at an early age to girls, drawing them in, selling them what they should look like—that is, what they should buy to look like the images.

Women's bodies are objects in our culture, used to uphold and impose impossible standards of beauty. There is no woman who is immune to this powerful psychological attack. So we have now created a culture in which women see their body as an object, too. Experts in women's health and body image issues see a literal separation between mind, body, and spirit, sometimes known as mind-body dualism. Read more about this dualism in the article "Out-of-Body Image," in *Ms.* magazine (Heldman 2008). It may help you understand why you or women you care about undergo plastic surgery, aggressive hair removal, Brazilian waxes, and other body-changing tactics. The factors that drive these feelings—that is, what makes the hair "unwanted"—is cultural.

WITHSTANDING CULTURAL INFLUENCES

> *I grew up in a very male-oriented household so I thought about how hard I could throw a ball, how fast I could swim, and how far I could run. I have never waxed or bleached or threaded and can't imagine the pain of having your hair ripped out.* —N.D.

Women's relationships with their body are complex. When we focus and rely on our body to empower us, it interferes with our real autonomy—the power to run our own lives. By diverting our attention away from leading a good and healthy life, and instead thinking about how to manipulate our bodies, we have lost many of our strengths as women. Instead of focusing outward, we focus inward. In "Out-of-Body Image," Caroline Heldman (2008) writes,

Unwanted Hair and Hirsutism

"Girls are taught: Your body is a project that needs work before you can attract others. Boys are taught: Your body is a tool to master the environment." Researchers and analysts suggest this is a deliberate ploy by the male-dominated society to distract us from the business of real liberation, which Gloria Steinem has said is a revolution, not public relations.

Social scientists theorize that males, unconsciously or consciously, feel threatened by women's power to create life and so try to control us in many ways, and thus have created the society described in these pages. Their most detrimental effort to control women's economic and emotional autonomy is to force women to carry a pregnancy, through legal action. When you think about it, why are so many men so hyped up about abortion? The pro-life movement, predominantly under the leadership of men, says it is about a baby and "life," but it is the life of the woman they are really focused on controlling and not toddlers or children they are protecting.

It is a struggle to make yourself immune to all these pressures, but it is worth it. The images and messages of how to be loved are very pervasive and invasive. We may not expect the knight in shining armor anymore, but we do want to be loved and accepted. Since much of our worth is invested in outer appearance (whether we admit it or not), feelings of self-loathing and low self-esteem are indeed driven by body image.

Unfortunately there's a lack of serious attention paid to unwanted hair by women's health-care providers. Make no mistake: unwanted hair is a very serious problem for at least 10 percent of the female population. Hirsutism significantly contributes to lower self-esteem and negative body image, which can predispose women to depression. Having some good information about how to cope with unwanted hair can help to empower more women and validate their experiences. But it is also important to look at our feelings about our unwanted hair and explore their origins.

Not all women with unwanted hair have a negative body image, but you may have a body image problem that warrants professional counseling if you are experiencing any of the following:

- Being preoccupied with your body hair
- Insisting you are too hairy when you have acceptable amounts of body hair (e.g., arms and pubic hair)
- Feeling guilty or ashamed to be seen in public

- Overly concerned about your appearance
- Experiencing noticeable mood changes in association with your appearance (e.g., self-loathing after trying on clothes in a store or looking in the mirror)
- Avoiding public, work, or family gatherings because you don't look good enough
- Not participating in activities that require you to wear shorts, bathing suits, and so on
- Avoiding sexual relations because you are ashamed of or hate your body

Read appendix A for some tips on overcoming obsession.

BODY HAIR ACTIVISM

If you are moved to take action and change the way you think about yourself and how society treats women, you are not alone. Thousands of women are waiting for you to join their ranks. Some women prefer to take personal steps, and others are energized by working with men and women who inspire and encourage them.

The Personal

You can feel more powerful and experience self-love by nurturing, protecting, and appreciating the body you were born with. It is an amazing creation—just look at how strong, resilient, and useful your hair is. See how it takes a chemical reaction brought on by an electrical current to kill a hair cell! It may take you awhile to love yourself and your hair, but if you try to nurture and protect yourself, self-love develops in time. What's great about it is that you don't need someone to love you first. In fact, once you love yourself, others will be drawn to you, wanting to experience some of that love.

The Buddhists believe that by loving yourself and exuding love you bring more love into the world—that you can change the world by how you treat yourself. Certainly, the world needs a lot of love. It is overwhelming to see the hardships suffered around the world, especially by women. As a comparison, see the extreme control of women forced to wear shrouds covering their body as soon as they hit puberty and those terminal hairs start to pop out. It's a horrendous form of social control, yet it is similar to controls in the United States and other "civilized" countries, only more extreme.

Unwanted Hair and Hirsutism

Think of the love a parent, guardian, or grandparent has showed you. If you are a mother, think of that complete, unconditional love you have for your child. Now, capture just a little of that love and adoration and wrap it around yourself. Nurture it. You are on your way to changing the world!

The Cultural

Artist and poet Robyn Levy created a cartoon starring Libby Doe who is a very hairy lady, and proud of it. She wrote a poem that begins, "I ain't no shave slave," articulating women's growing frustration with feeling culturally pressed to remove body hair. In protest, Levy keeps her body hair intact. There are many women like Levy, who do not shave and go all natural all the time.

In fact, European women are far less likely to be "shave slaves" than are North American women. Compare them to us. Are they loved less? Have less romantic partners? Get married less? Absolutely not. Logic will tell you that our cultural obsession with hairless women has not a hair to stand on.

One compelling example of body hair activism comes from a New York performance artist named Jennifer Miller, director of an alternative circus-theater company called Circus Amok. Miller has facial hair growth that is extensive enough for her to have a full moustache and beard, but her line of work makes it possible for her to go natural. Miller has worn her facial hair intact for many years, and rejects societal and cultural pressure to "correct" her facial hair growth daily. Miller admits that she certainly would not have chosen to have a beard, and has endured humiliation and public displays of outrage over her appearance. Nevertheless, at the same time she feels that her beard is her identity; it is part of who she is. Miller's courage to display her facial hair is a personal act of protest that is very political. Perhaps this woman's courage, like that of so many, may help to dispel the stigma and myths associated with hirsutism.

The Political

There are groups of women who are so fed up with the hairless standard that they are saying, "NO MORE!" The Gorilla Girls was an inspiring group that spawned activist groups all over the country in the 1980s and 1990s. Although hair removal wasn't their reason for being, just as it's not for feminist activist groups active today, it is part of the larger movement to change society's culture and to liberate women.

There are many international nonprofits that work to educate and protect women, both in this hemisphere and around the world. Notable ones in the United States are the Feminist Majority Foundation, CARE, National Organization for Women, and NARAL Pro-Choice America.

Some early evidence indicates that increased levels of hormones in the environment are causing biological changes in women's bodies. Women have more fat and fat repositories (breasts, for example) where hormones are aggregating. Some believe this is causing earlier puberty in women and a rise in various cancers. Certainly hormonal changes are related to hirsutism and PCOS as described earlier. You can become involved in movements to protect consumers through transparent food labeling, regulating pesticides and hormones used in agriculture, and the "seed" movement (preventing conglomerate companies from "owning" a seed used for food throughout the world). The Center for Science in the Public Interest (CSPI) is one group lobbying for consumer protection. You can sign up for its newsletter at www.cspinet.org, which alerts readers about unhealthy food widely available in supermarkets.

Unwanted Hair and Hirsutism

The Personal Is Political

> *Leg hair, well, I let it grow on and off in the 1960s and 1970s, which was probably one of my worst fashion decisions. It was uneven and weird: not much on the knees, sparse around the ankles, and real furry elsewhere. What was I thinking? Now, armpit hair, that was better, a nice pelt, I thought, though it probably grossed out a lot of people. Too bad, I liked it. The leg hair wasn't so satisfying as a fashion statement, though it probably worked as a "fuck you" statement.*
>
> *The big bush, I always liked that. But I didn't like that it grew way the hell down my legs. When I wasn't shaving it was a major statement wearing shorts. I'm still lazy and only shave in the summer or when I am lap swimming. But the bush I wouldn't shave, not even when men I liked gave in to shameless begging.* —P.A.

If you are a teenager or preteen reading this book, now is the time to consider going au naturel, or at least bleaching; once you start the hair removal process, it is tough to go back. Perhaps if you must try to remove hair from one area, choose your underarms. It is a small space to deal with the rest of your life.

If you are berated by peers, you can laugh all the way to the bank as you save tons of money and time; soon you will learn time is money. And who knows, you might start a trend!

APPENDIX A

CAN'T STOP OBSESSING

Once your mind gets hooked on an obsession, it is hard to let go. It might be that unwanted hair above your lip, under your belly button, or on your arms you constantly see or feel that gets you hooked. You might be obsessing about your hair to take your mind off a bigger problem. Whatever the case may be, it might be time to reach out to friends, family, or a professional to support you while you sift through and go after what is bothering you.

Maybe you obsess because you don't like your body; if that is the case, there are ways to retrain your mind. First, take a break from mainstream and entertainment-oriented media. Then sign up for a yoga class, personal training, a movement class, or some other body-centered activity with a sensitive trainer. These healthy distractions can help you gently and personally learn more about and feel comfortable with your body.

Are you obsessing because you are too centered on yourself? Are you always worried what others think about you? Are you self-conscious? Shy? Get involved in activities that make the world a better place. What topics interest you? Help relieve your pain and suffering as well as that of others by simply getting involved. Volunteer opportunities abound for groups dedicated to protecting and improving the lives of women and girls, as do groups advocating for civil, environmental, and health rights and causes of all kinds. Once you feel engaged and committed to other causes, the hair you hate won't seem so important.

Or maybe you're not centered enough on yourself. Are you a caregiver who is always thinking about what others' need? Women are often taking care of children, partners, a disabled loved one, grandchildren, siblings, or parents—or several generations at the same time. It is easy to obsess about your body, which is right in front of you at all times, when you don't have the opportunity to be involved in other activities that you might enjoy. It is like getting caught up in the minutia of planning three meals a day, every day. You see those same hairs day after day. Get involved in a support group that offers a diversion and resources, if not outright substitute care from a caregiver service. In between meetings, read caregiver Web sites for tips, empathy, and encouragement, and write blogs sharing your own experiences.

Are you reacting to negative comments by a partner, family member, or friend? Ongoing, harsh insults are abusive and you should seek help to stop them or remove yourself from the situation. During occasional criticisms and mean jokes, tell yourself immediately that person's opinion doesn't count and he or she is not your judge. Try to focus on something you like about yourself while this is happening. If you can, confront the person criticizing your hair or body, and ask him or her to stop. If the other person does not stop, say, "Well, I like my [adjective] hair and body," and walk away or change the subject. Find courage by practicing to yourself or in your journal.

All of these suggestions might be a major change for you, and change can provoke anxiety. It is hard to know what to do and what to expect. Unless you want things to stay the same without any hope of relief, you must suffer through a little anxiety along the way to realize the benefits.

APPENDIX B

COMMON PRESCRIPTION DRUGS THAT MAY CAUSE HAIR GROWTH

Some of the following drugs can cause hair growth at certain doses, particularly oral contraceptives (OCs), which are also used to limit hair growth. Your doctor or an endocrinologist should explore any side effects you are experiencing. There could be a similar drug that does not activate your hair growth but has the same benefits, which is particularly true of OCs.

Type of Drug	Typically Used For
Some selective serotonin uptake inhibitors (e.g., Prozac, Serafem, or Paxil) and some serotonin-norepinephrine reuptake inhibitors (e.g., Effexor)	Mild to moderate depression, major depression, PMS
Combination oral contraceptives that contain one of two synthetic estrogens (ethinyl estradiol or mestranol) and one of 12 progestins (e.g., norethindrone; norethindrone acetate; Endometriosis ethynodiol diacetate; morethynodrel; levonorgestrel; dl-norgestrel; norgesteimate; desogestrel; gestodene; chloramdinone acetate; megestrol acetate; medoroxyprogesterone acetate)	Birth control, cycle control, PMS, polycystic ovarian syndrome (PCOS)
Progestin-only contraceptives e.g., Injections of Depo Provera (depot medroxyprogesterone acetate); implants such as Norplant, Ortho Evra patch, some OC pills	Birth control
Progestins (see list of progestins under combination oral contraceptives)	Menstrual cycle control, prevents early miscarriage in pregnancy, shedding the uterine lining when there is too much lining (endometrial hyperplasia)

Unwanted Hair and Hirsutism

Type of Drug	Typically Used For
Hormone replacement therapy (contains synthetic estrogens and progestins; see list under combination OC)	Replacing lost estrogen after menopause to protect against postmenopausal heart disease, osteoporosis, and menopausal discomforts
Corticosteroids	Allergies, inflammatory conditions such as Crohn's disease
Diuretics	Fluid retention
Oral hypoglycemic agents	Type 2 diabetes or impaired glucose tolerance, polycystic ovarian syndrome (PCOS)
Anticonvulsants	Seizures

Source: International Hair Route Drug Chart: List of Proprietary Drugs Which Name Hirsutism as a Possible Side Effect, International Hair Route *(December 2000). For the updated list, visit www.hairroute.com.*

APPENDIX C

ORAL CONTRACEPTION

ESTROGEN VERSUS PROGESTIN: SIDE EFFECTS

Many of the side effects you may experience on oral contraception are dose related. In other words, if you go on a lower-dose contraceptive, your side effects will likely disappear. In some cases, you may even require a slightly higher-dose contraceptive—particularly if you have a history of heavy uterine bleeding.

The good news is that if you are experiencing androgenic side effects, it is very easy to fix. Simply request a low-dose, triphasic OC with a low-activity selective progestin, which, studies show, make a difference in reducing side effects.

DIFFERENT BODIES NEED DIFFERENT ORAL CONTRACEPTIVES

- If you have tender breasts, heavy periods, and clots, request a low-estrogen, full-progestin OC, which will bring your cycles under control.
- If you have acne, oily skin, unwanted hair in places other than the underarms and legs, or if you suffer from PMS and mood swings, request a low-progestin OC.
- If you're not getting your period on your OC, this is a sign that you need a low-progestin OC.
- If you have been unable to tolerate a combination OC, you may want to request an extremely low-dose OC, which delivers lower doses of both estrogen and progestin.
- Although migraine sufferers are on the "stay away from OC" list, it is important to note that when it comes to migraines, the side effects vary. In fact, about 33 percent of women on an OC will notice an improvement in migraine headaches; 33 percent will notice no change at all; wheareas another 33 percent will notice that their migraines get worse, which means that for them, the OC is not a good choice. Progestin-only pills are good alternatives.

Unwanted Hair and Hirsutism

- If you have heart disease or a heart condition, use a progestin-only pill.
- If you're diabetic, stay on top of your blood sugar levels. OCs can actually alter your insulin requirements because the progestins used in combination OCs can decrease glucose tolerance and increase insulin resistance.
- If you have high blood pressure and decide to go on an OC, have your blood pressure checked every three months during your first year.

BIBLIOGRAPHY

"AACE Hyperandrogenism Guidelines," American Association of Clinical Endocrinologists Medical Guidelines for Clinical Practice for the Diagnosis and Treatment of Hyperandrogenic Disorders. *Endocrine Practice* 7, no. 2 (March/April 2001).

"AEA Laser Position Statement: FDA Clearance of Laser Hair Removal Devices." Revised August 2000. American Electrology Association, htttp://www.electrology.com.

American Academy of Dermatology, htttp://www.aad.org (June 2008).

"American Association of Clinical Endocrinologists Medical Guidelines for Clinical Practice for the Diagnosis and Treatment of Hyperandrogenic Disorders." *Endocrine Practice* 7, no. 2 (March/April 2001).

American Electrology Association, http://www.electrology.com (May 15, 2008).

American Medical Media, *Hair Removal Journal*, http://www.hairremovaljournal.org (May 2008).

Androgen Excess Society, http://www.androgenexcesssociety.org (May 15, 2008).

Ashack, Richard J., M.D. "Psoriasis and Electrology: An Overview." *Perspectives* (Spring/Summer, 1996).

Azziz, Ricardo, M.D., M.P.H. "Current Hormonal Therapy of Androgen Excess." International Hair Route, http://www.hairroute.com (December 2000).

———. "Hirsutism and Androgen Excess: Defining the Problem." The Society of Clinical and Medical Electrologists, http://www.scmeweb.org (December 2000).

———. "Shaving and Hirsutism: Does It Make It Worse?" The Society of Clinical and Medical Electrologists, http://www.scmeweb.org (December 2000).

Bell, Ruth, ed. *Changing Bodies, Changing Lives*, 3rd ed. (New York: Times Books, 1998).

Bono, Michael. "The Michael Bono Series: The Infundibulum." http://www.electrology.com (December 2000).

———. "The Michael Bono Series: The Macrophage." http://www.electrology.com (December 2000).

Boston Women's Health Book Collective. *Our Bodies, Ourselves: A New Edition for a New Era* (New York: Simon & Schuster, Inc., 2005).

Boston Women's Health Book Collective, http://www.ourbodiesourselves.org (May 2008).

CARES Foundation, http://www.caresfoundation.org (May 2008).

Carter, J. J., and S. W. Lanigan. "Incidence of Acne from Reactions after Laser Hair Removal." *Lasers in Medical Science* (London: Springer-Verlag, Ltd., 2006).

"CBC-TV Probes Laser Hair Removal." International Hair Route, http://www.hairroute.com (December 2000).

Chinnappa, Priya, M.D., and Adi Mehta, M.D. "Hirsutism." http://www.clevelandclinicmeded.com/medicalpubs (February 13, 2004).

Chrousos, G. P., M.D., FAAP, MACP, MACEMD, MACE. "Glucocorticoid Therapy and Cushing Syndrome." http://www.emedicine.com (June 23, 2006).

Copperthwaite, Derek R. "Editorial." International Hair Route, http://www.hairroute.com (May 24, 2000).

Corn Is King, by filmmakers Aaron Woolf, Curt Ellis, and Ian Cheney, a coproduction of Mosaic Films Incorporated and the Independent Television Service, http://www.pbs.org/independentlens/kingcorn (2006).

Deplewski, Diane, and Robert L. Rosenfield. "Role of Hormones in Pilosebaceous Unit Development." *Endocrine Reviews* 21, no. 4 (2000): 363–92.

Dumesic, Daniel A., M.D., and Rebekah R. Herrmann. "Estimated Prevalence of Undiagnosed Glucose Intolerance from Androgenic

Anovulation Among Women Requesting Electrolysis." The Society of Clinical and Medical Electrologists, htttp://www.scmeweb.org (December 2000).

Elder, Stacey A. "After-Electrolysis Skincare." International Hair Route, http://www.hairroute.com (May 24, 2000).

Electrology, http://www.electrology.com (March 2008).

"EMLA: An Educational File." International Hair Route, http://www.hairroute.com (December 2000).

"Evaluation and Treatment of Hirsutism in Premenopausal Women: An Endocrine Society Clinical Practice Guideline." *The Journal of Clinical Endocrinology & Metabolism* 93, no. 4 (2000): 1105–20.

Farid, Nadir R., M.D., and Norene Gilletz. *The PCOS Diet Cookbook: Easy and Delicious Recipes & Tips for Women with PCOS on the Low GI Diet* (Lexington, KY: Your Health Press, 2007).

Ferriman, D. M., and J. D. Gallwey. *Journal of Clinical Endocrinology & Metabolism* (1961): 1442–43.

"General and Plastic Surgery Devices: Reclassification of the Tweezer-Type Epilator." A publication of the Department of Health and Human Services, Food and Drug Administration [Docket No. 97N4199].

Goldberg, David, M.D., J.D. "Legal Issues in Laser Operation." *Clinics in Dermatology* 24, no. 1 (January–February 2006): 56–59.

Greenblatt, Robert B., M.D. "Hair Growth: The Role of Heredity, Genetics, and Androgenic Metabolism." *Journal of Electrology*, http://www.electrology.com (December 2000).

Griffing, George T., M.D. "Hirsutism." eMedicine, http://www.WebMd.com (October 12, 2007).

Hair Facts, http://www.hairfacts.com (May 2008).

Hair There and Everywhere. Documentary. Aired on CBC Newsworld (May 15, 2001).

Hanley, H. Christina, M.D. "Hirsutism: Causes and Treatment." *Journal of Electrology*, http://www.electrology.com (December 2000).

Heldman, Caroline, "Out-of-Body Image." *Ms.* (Spring 2008).

"Hirsutism, and the Variety of Human Perspectives." International Hair Route, http://www.hairroute.com (May 24, 2000).

"International Hair Route Drug Chart: List of Proprietary Drugs Which Name Hirsutism as a Possible Side Effect." International Hair Route, http://www.hairroute.com (December 2000).

Institute Research Associates, htttp://www.consumerlaserguide.com (May 2008).

James, Andrea. "Blinded by the Light." American Electrology Association, http://www.electrology.com (April 1999).

Katz, Eugene, M.D. "Hirsutism." *Journal of Electrology,* htttp://www.electrology.com (December 2000).

Keratin.com, http://www.keratin.com (July 2008).

"Laser Hair Removal: Current Findings with the Long Pulse Ruby Laser." The Society of Clinical and Medical Electrologists, http://www.scmeweb.org (December 1997).

Laser Hair Removal Consumer Guide (Los Angeles: Institute of Laser Medicine, 2007).

Lazerblazers, http://www.laserblazers.com (May 2008).

Legro, Richard, M.D. "Hirsutism: Etiology and Treatment." *The Female Patient* 27 (October 2002).

Mastroianni, Anna C., Ruth Faden, and Daniel Federman, eds. *Women and Health Research: Ethical and Legal Issues of Including Women in Clinical Studies,* vol. 1 (Washington: National Academy Press, 1994).

Mayo Foundation for Medical Education and Research (MFMER), http://www.mayoclinic.com/health/laser-hair-removal/HQ00981 (March 28, 2008).

McAleer, Sally, C.P.E. "Public Relations and the American Electrology Association." http://www.electrology.com (December 2000).

Meharg, G. E., M.D., and R. N. Richards, M.D. "Cosmetic and Medical Electrolysis and Temporary Hair Removal: A Practical Manual and Reference Guide." http://www.electrology.com (December 2000).

Molczan, Ted. "Permanent Hair Reduction: A Legal Pandora's Box." American Electrology Association, http://www.electrology.com (December 2000).

———. "Permanent Hair Removal Using Microwaves?" *Electrology World* (Summer 1998).

New Zealand Dermatological Society Incorporated, http://www.dermnetnz.org (November 2008)

Owens, Shelby, C.C.E. "The Integumentary System." The Society of Clinical and Medical Electrologists, http://www.scmeweb.org (Winter 1996).

"PCOS," http://www.DiagnoseMeFirst.com (June 12, 2008).

Petricca, Teresa E., C.P.E. "We Must Maintain Our Unique Selling Position." *Electrology World* (Winter 1999).

Polycystic Ovarian Syndrome Association, Inc., http://www.pcosupport.org (June 12, 2008).

Redd, Nancy Amanda. *Body Drama* (New York: Gotham Books, 2008).

Redmond, Geoffrey P., M.D. "Endocrine Perspective." International Hair Route, http://www.hairroute.com (May 24, 2000).

Rosenthal, M. Sara. *Women and Unwanted Hair* (Toronto: Your Health Press, 2001).

Sahoo, Alison. "The Diode Laser for Hair Removal: The Next Generation in Laser Treatment." *Perspectives* (Spring/Summer 1998).

Schuster, James, M.D. "Pregnancy," http://www.electrology.com. (December 2000).

Sherwin, Susan. *No Longer Patient: Feminist Ethics & Health Care* (Philadelphia: Temple University Press, 1992).

"Skin Talk." International Hair Route, http://www.hairroute.com (December 2000).

U.S. National Library of Medicine, http://www.ncbi.nlm.nih.gov/pubmed (May 2008).

INDEX

A
alopecia, 31–33, 40, 50, 72–73, 99
anagen, 27–28, 93, 125, 131, 138
androgens, 30–33, 40–41, 50–55, 61, 67–68. 73, 83, 86–90
anorexia nervosa, 23, 41, 55
antiandrogen creams, 66
antiandrogens, 65, 67
apocrine glands, 24
axillary hair, 33
axillary region, 40

B
belly button/happy trail, 113
bleaching cream, 100
Brazilian bikini wax, 118

C
carcinogenic, 130
catagen, 27–28, 125, 138
catecholamines, 54
Certified Medical Electrologist (CME), 136
Certified Professional Electrologist (CPE), 136
CLHRP—Certified Laser Hair Removal Professional, 148
Compendium of Pharmaceuticals and Specialties (CPS), 51
Consumer Guide to Laser Hair Removal, 139
contact dermatitis, 97, 99
corticosteroid, 83
Cushing's syndrome, 46, 49–50, 55, 67
cyproterone acetate, 61, 66

D
depilation, 86
dermal papilla, 25–28, 85, 125
dermis, 26
diabetes, 33, 46, 51–52, 67, 72–73, 76–77, 82–83, 122–23, 162
dihydrotestosterone, 33
diuretic, 162
drospirenone, 66

E
eflornithine, 58, 68, 99
eflornithine hydrochloride, 68, 99
electric tweezer, 95
electrologist, 48. 93, 125–37, 149
electrolysis, 26–27, 87, 91, 96, 106, 125–33, 136, 166–68
endocrinologist, 31–32, 38, 44–50, 56–62, 68, 70, 93, 106, 161
epidermis, 25–26, 86
epilation, 15–16, 86–87, 96–97, 115, 134
epilators, 96–97
estrogen, 60–62, 77–79, 160–63
eyebrow shaping, 108

F
Federal Drug Administration (FDA), 58, 69–70, 89–90, 94, 99, 105, 126, 140–42, 144, 147–50, 165
federal regulations, 147
Ferriman-Gallwey index, 43
finasteride, 66
fingers, 113
5-alpha-reductase, 33, 66
flutamide, 66
focal hirsutism, 38–39, 44–45

170

folliculitis, 17–18, 87, 92–93, 96, 102, 125, 129
40-Year-Old Virgin, 19
friction, 101

G
galvanic current, 128
glucocorticoids, 67
glycemic index (GI), 75
GnRH agonist, 68
gonadotropin releasing hormones (GnRH), 68
growth inhibiting creams, 99

H
hair follicle, 15–16, 22–33, 69, 85–87, 99–104, 125–29, 138–39, 143
hair removal cream, 97–98, 114
hair root, 85
hair shaft, 17, 25–27, 33, 86, 90, 97, 125, 138, 144
hirsutism, 13–14, 22–23, 30–33, 37–73, 76, 78, 87–92, 97, 100, 128, 134–35, 156–57
HIV, 128, 144
home electrolysis kits, 104
hyperandrogenic insulin-resistant acanthosis nigricans (HAIRAN syndrome), 53
hyperandrogenic syndrome, 40
hyperandrogenism, 33, 60, 68
hyperthyroidism, 41
hypertrichosis, 23, 41–42, 49, 87

I J
idiopathic hirsutism, 39, 47, 56–58
ingrown hair, 17–18, 87, 92, 95
insulin resistance, 51

K
keloids, 17, 87
keratin, 25, 28, 97, 168

L
lanugo hair, 24
laser hair removal, 106, 138, 145, 150
laser razor, 94
libido, 30–31, 64

M
melanin, 138–139, 142
melanocytes, 24
menopause, 17, 31–32, 40, 61, 65, 86–88, 122, 162
metabolism, 33, 48
mind-body dualism, 153

N
Nonclassic congenital adrenal hyperplasia (NCAH), 52

O
obesity, 54
oral contraceptives, 60, 63–64, 67, 163
Our Bodies, Ourselves: A New Edition for a New Era, 12

P
PCOS Diet Cookbook, 74, 82
Physician's Desk Reference, 50
pilosebaceous unit, 33, 40
Premenstrual syndrome (PMS), 62–63, 161–63
polycystic ovarian syndrome (PCOS), 39, 44–46, 49, 53, 55, 58–60, 67, 71–79, 83–83, 157, 161–62, 167
polycystic ovary, 75

porphyria, 41
pregnancy, 31–33, 40, 46, 56, 60–62, 73, 84–88, 123, 154, 161
prescription drugs that may cause hair growth, 161–62
progestin, 60–68, 84, 160–63
pubic hair, 118–24

R
romaraji, 13

S
sebaceous gland, 33
seborrhea, 40
sebum, 24
Sex and the City, 118
shaving, 18, 91–94, 115–17, 143, 165
skin appendage, 23
spironolactone, 66
Stein-Leventhal syndrome, 71
stress, 54–55, 68, 79
subcutaneous tissue layer, 26
sugaring, 101

T
telogen, 27–28, 125, 138
terminal hair, 24–35, 38–46, 56–59, 86–88, 98
ThermoLase, 141–42
thermolysis, 127
threading, 102
toes, 113
topical analgesic, 129
topical anesthetic, 142
trimmers, 94
tumors, 55
tweezing, 95

U
Ugly Betty, 14
Uniprobe Electolysis Probe, 128

V
Vaniqa, 69, 99–100
vellus hair, 16, 24–28, 31–35, 39–40, 97–98, 127
vulvitis, 121–22

W
waxing, 103, 109, 116, 121

X
X-ray, 144

Y Z
yeast infections, 122

Printed in Great Britain
by Amazon.co.uk, Ltd.,
Marston Gate.